A complete practice of midwifery Consisting of upwards of forty cases or observations in that valuable art, selected from many others, in the course of a very extensive practice Recommended to all female practitioners in an art so importan

Sarah Stone

A complete practice of midwifery. Consisting of upwards of forty cases or observations in that valuable art, selected from many others, in the course of a very extensive practice. ... Recommended to all female practitioners in an art so important to the lives and well-being of the sex. By Sarah Stone, ...
Stone, Sarah
ESTCID: T163353
Reproduction from Countway Library of Medicine
With a half-title.
London : printed for T. Cooper, 1737.
xxxii,113,118-163,[1]p. ; 8°

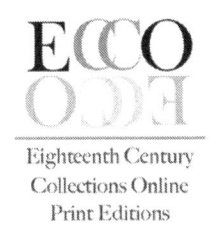

Eighteenth Century Collections Online Print Editions

Gale ECCO Print Editions

Relive history with *Eighteenth Century Collections Online*, now available in print for the independent historian and collector. This series includes the most significant English-language and foreign-language works printed in Great Britain during the eighteenth century, and is organized in seven different subject areas including literature and language; medicine, science, and technology; and religion and philosophy. The collection also includes thousands of important works from the Americas.

The eighteenth century has been called "The Age of Enlightenment." It was a period of rapid advance in print culture and publishing, in world exploration, and in the rapid growth of science and technology – all of which had a profound impact on the political and cultural landscape. At the end of the century the American Revolution, French Revolution and Industrial Revolution, perhaps three of the most significant events in modern history, set in motion developments that eventually dominated world political, economic, and social life.

In a groundbreaking effort, Gale initiated a revolution of its own: digitization of epic proportions to preserve these invaluable works in the largest online archive of its kind. Contributions from major world libraries constitute over 175,000 original printed works. Scanned images of the actual pages, rather than transcriptions, recreate the works ***as they first appeared.***

Now for the first time, these high-quality digital scans of original works are available via print-on-demand, making them readily accessible to libraries, students, independent scholars, and readers of all ages.

For our initial release we have created seven robust collections to form one the world's most comprehensive catalogs of 18th century works.

Initial Gale ECCO Print Editions collections include:

> ***History and Geography***
> Rich in titles on English life and social history, this collection spans the world as it was known to eighteenth-century historians and explorers. Titles include a wealth of travel accounts and diaries, histories of nations from throughout the world, and maps and charts of a world that was still being discovered. Students of the War of American Independence will find fascinating accounts from the British side of conflict.

Social Science
Delve into what it was like to live during the eighteenth century by reading the first-hand accounts of everyday people, including city dwellers and farmers, businessmen and bankers, artisans and merchants, artists and their patrons, politicians and their constituents. Original texts make the American, French, and Industrial revolutions vividly contemporary.

Medicine, Science and Technology
Medical theory and practice of the 1700s developed rapidly, as is evidenced by the extensive collection, which includes descriptions of diseases, their conditions, and treatments. Books on science and technology, agriculture, military technology, natural philosophy, even cookbooks, are all contained here.

Literature and Language
Western literary study flows out of eighteenth-century works by Alexander Pope, Daniel Defoe, Henry Fielding, Frances Burney, Denis Diderot, Johann Gottfried Herder, Johann Wolfgang von Goethe, and others. Experience the birth of the modern novel, or compare the development of language using dictionaries and grammar discourses.

Religion and Philosophy
The Age of Enlightenment profoundly enriched religious and philosophical understanding and continues to influence present-day thinking. Works collected here include masterpieces by David Hume, Immanuel Kant, and Jean-Jacques Rousseau, as well as religious sermons and moral debates on the issues of the day, such as the slave trade. The Age of Reason saw conflict between Protestantism and Catholicism transformed into one between faith and logic -- a debate that continues in the twenty-first century.

Law and Reference
This collection reveals the history of English common law and Empire law in a vastly changing world of British expansion. Dominating the legal field is the *Commentaries of the Law of England* by Sir William Blackstone, which first appeared in 1765. Reference works such as almanacs and catalogues continue to educate us by revealing the day-to-day workings of society.

Fine Arts
The eighteenth-century fascination with Greek and Roman antiquity followed the systematic excavation of the ruins at Pompeii and Herculaneum in southern Italy; and after 1750 a neoclassical style dominated all artistic fields. The titles here trace developments in mostly English-language works on painting, sculpture, architecture, music, theater, and other disciplines. Instructional works on musical instruments, catalogs of art objects, comic operas, and more are also included.

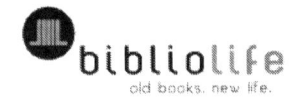

The BiblioLife Network

This project was made possible in part by the BiblioLife Network (BLN), a project aimed at addressing some of the huge challenges facing book preservationists around the world. The BLN includes libraries, library networks, archives, subject matter experts, online communities and library service providers. We believe every book ever published should be available as a high-quality print reproduction; printed on-demand anywhere in the world. This insures the ongoing accessibility of the content and helps generate sustainable revenue for the libraries and organizations that work to preserve these important materials.

The following book is in the "public domain" and represents an authentic reproduction of the text as printed by the original publisher. While we have attempted to accurately maintain the integrity of the original work, there are sometimes problems with the original work or the micro-film from which the books were digitized. This can result in minor errors in reproduction. Possible imperfections include missing and blurred pages, poor pictures, markings and other reproduction issues beyond our control. Because this work is culturally important, we have made it available as part of our commitment to protecting, preserving, and promoting the world's literature.

GUIDE TO FOLD-OUTS MAPS and OVERSIZED IMAGES

The book you are reading was digitized from microfilm captured over the past thirty to forty years. Years after the creation of the original microfilm, the book was converted to digital files and made available in an online database.

In an online database, page images do not need to conform to the size restrictions found in a printed book. When converting these images back into a printed bound book, the page sizes are standardized in ways that maintain the detail of the original. For large images, such as fold-out maps, the original page image is split into two or more pages

Guidelines used to determine how to split the page image follows:

• Some images are split vertically; large images require vertical and horizontal splits.
• For horizontal splits, the content is split left to right.
• For vertical splits, the content is split from top to bottom.
• For both vertical and horizontal splits, the image is processed from top left to bottom right.

A

Complete Practice

OF

MIDWIFERY.

A Complete Practice

OF

MIDWIFERY.

Consisting of

Upwards of FORTY CASES or OBSERVATIONS in that valuable ART, selected from many Others, in the Course of a very EXTENSIVE PRACTICE.

And Interspersed

With many necessary CAUTIONS and useful INSTRUCTIONS, proper to be observed in the most Dangerous and Critical Exigencies, as well when the Delivery is difficult in its own Nature, as when it becomes so by the Rashness or Ignorance of Unexperienc'd Pretenders.

Recommended to

All FEMALE PRACTITIONERS in an Art so important to the LIVES and WELL-BEING of the SEX

By *SARAH STONE*,
Of PICCADILLY.

LONDON.
Printed for T COOPER, at the *Globe* in *Pater-Noster Row.* MDCCXXXVII

TO THE

QUEEN's
Moſt Excellent Majeſty.

MADAM,

FORGIVE my preſuming to approach YOUR MAJESTY with the following Sheets; a liberty I ſhould not dare to take with the greateſt of Queens, was I not at the ſame time encouraged by that Univerſal Benevolence, which ſtiles You the Nursing-mother of a most happy people.

Your Majesty's tender regard to our Sex's modesty, makes a Treatise of Midwifery implore Your Royal Protection; the practice of which is generally so little understood by Women Midwives, especially in the Country: where tho' the Women are commonly more robust, and pure Nature in great measure assists, the least difficulty has frequently baffled the Midwife's judgment, and she often forced to send for a Man; when the Labour has been no more than a common Case, as a Child's pitching wrong, &c. And

DEDICATION.

And there's another misfortune, that 'tis rare to find in the Country, Gentlemen that are grave and old experienc'd Practitioners; which forces our Sex to submit to every boyish Pretender; by which our modesty is exposed, and the Midwife's reputation hurt: to prevent which (as far as in my power) I resolv'd to publish some Observations in my Practice; in hopes they'll prove instructive to some Women Midwives, especially those of the lower class. And in this undertaking, to whom can I fly for Protection, but to YOUR MAJESTY, the Fountain of all perfect Virtue,

viii DEDICATION.

tue, and the generous Encourager of all Arts and Sciences.

I will not venture to touch on YOUR MAJESTY's Excellencies; that many learned pens have tried, and all fell infinitely short of: and therefore must unwillingly be silent where I ought to express most; and, imploring YOUR MAJESTY's Royal Protection and Forgiveness, beg leave to subscribe myself,

YOUR MAJESTY's

Most Obedient, and most

Humbly Devoted Servant,

Sarah Stone.

THE PREFACE TO THE READER.

THE Occasion of my publishing this small Treatise is, in hopes it may prove instructive to some Women Professors in the Art of Midwifery; and inform them in a right, safe, and just practice of that Art: that they may be able to deliver in difficult Labours, as well as those that are not so. For I cannot

cannot comprehend, why Women are not capable of compleating this business when begun, without calling in of Men to their assistance, who are often sent for, when the Work is near finish'd; and then the Midwife, who has taken all the pains, is accounted of little value, and the young men command all the praise. Which unskilful practices of Women-Midwives being often repeated, give occasion for Pregnant Women to bespeak them, so that it is become quite a fashion; especially with the *Bristol* Ladies.

I am well assured, unless the Women-Midwives give themselves more to the Study of this Art, and learn the difficult part of their business, that the Modesty of our Sex will be in great danger of being lost, for want

want of good Women-Midwives, by being so much exposed to the Men professing this Art: for 'tis arrived to that height already, that almost every young Man, who hath served his Apprenticeship to a Barber-Surgeon, immediately sets up for a Man-Midwife; altho' as ignorant, and, indeed, much ignoranter, than the meanest Woman of the Profession.

But these young Gentlemen-Professors put on a finish'd assurance, with pretence that their Knowledge exceeds any Woman's, because they have seen, or gone thro', a Course of Anatomy: and so, if the Mother, or Child, or both die, as it often happens, then they die *Secundum Artem*; for a Man was there, and the Woman-Midwife bears all the blame. Then it is, that

that our young and well-assur'd pretenders boast, had they been there soon, neither should have died. Tho' I have made it my Observation within these few years, That more Women and Children have died by the hands of such Professors, than by the greatest imbecillity and ignorance of some Women-Midwives, who never went thro', or so much as heard of, a Course of Anatomy. For, give me leave to tell those young Gentlemen pretenders, who undertake the Practice of Midwifery with only the knowledge of dissecting the Dead, that all the Living who have or shall come under their care, in any difficulty, have and may severely pay for what knowledge they attain to in the Art of Midwifery; especially such young ones as now pretend to practise: by by whom (I am well assured) there are many sufferers both Mothers and Children; yea, Infants have been born alive, with their Brains working out of their Heads: occasion'd by the too common use of Instruments: which I never found but very little use to be made of, in all my practice. I have had the opportunity of going thro' a great number of difficult Labours, living in and near *Taunton*, a place where there was no Man-Midwife, and a town wholly depending on the Woollen Manufactory, the Combing and Weaving Part, which many Women are bred to there; and, I believe, has been the occasion of many Wrong Births and Bad Labours, which I was obliged to be at, among the poorer sort of Women. And as I never found

found Instruments requisite above four times in my life; so I am certain, where twenty Women are deliver'd with Instruments (which is now become a common practice) that nineteen of them might be deliver'd without, if not the twentieth, as will appear in my Observations. Wherefore it is my intention (with God's assistance) to instruct my Sisters of the Profession; that it may be in their power to deliver all manner of Births, with more ease and safety, than has hitherto been practis'd by many of them, and without exposing the Lives of their Women and Children to every boyish Pretender. For dissecting the Dead, and being just and tender to the Living, are vastly different; for it must be supposed that there is a tender regard one Woman bears

bears to another, and a natural Sympathy in those that have gone thro' the Pangs of Childbearing; which, doubtless, occasion a compassion for those that labour under those circumstances, which no man can be a judge of.

I have seen several Women open'd; and 'tis not improper for all of the Profession to see Dissections, and read Anatomy, as I have done. But had I inspected into them all my life, and not been instructed in Midwifery by my Mother, and Deputy to her full six years, it would have signified but little; nor should I have dared to have undertaken such a Profession, lest any Life should have been lost thro' my ignorance; which I am well assured, thro' the blessing of God, has never happened.

pened. I am not in the least condemning just Practitioners, men of erudition, grave and sedate, and whose judgments are unquestionable: they, without doubt, are justly to be esteem'd. But my whole design in this small piece is to be plain in my instructions, that Midwives of the lowest capacity may be able to Deliver their Women, without calling in, or sending for, a Man, in every little seeming difficulty; but if they have not strength, which I take to be the occasion of requiring their assistance in some circumstances; I would advise the Midwives of *Bristol*, to take special care to send for a just Practitioner; and, if possible, one without partiality: who values a Mother's and Child's Life, and the Midwife's Reputation,

tation, more than his own sinister Ends.

In my humble opinion, it is necessary that Midwives should employ three years at least, with some ingenious woman practising this Art. For if seven years must be served to learn a Trade, I think three years as little as possible to be instructed in an Art where Life depends.

I believe I shall make it appear, that a great part of the Miscarriage of many Midwives, occasioning the sufferings of several Mothers and Children, is for want of knowledge when to assist a Woman, and when to omit it. I have often been call'd to the assistance of many Midwives, and have found Mothers and Children in the utmost danger; which has been by begining

ing their work before its due time; they imagining every uncertain Pain a Woman hath, to be her Labour: which Pains are common, and attend many Women a Month or Six Weeks before their Time of Delivery (which I have found by experience.)

I shall not fill any part of this book, with needless discourses on the Parts of Generation, nor the Reasons of Conception; neither shall I concern myself, or give my opinion, why some Women do not conceive; many Authors being copious on such Subjects. For my part, I think all the Disorders of Teeming Women do not belong to Midwives; but they ought to commit themselves to the Care of a Physician; a Midwife's business

ness being only to be well instructed in her Profession: then with a good Resolution, and the Blessing of God, she needs not fear going thro' the most difficult part of her business, with as good success as I have done these five and thirty years. For I am well assured, that abundance of hard Labours are owing to the want of good judgment in the first beginnings of Travail.

Excuse me if I have been guilty of Prolixity, Tautology, or Circumlocution; my design in this Treatise being to instruct the meanest capacity, and not to meddle with those of Erudition, &c. I heartily wish what I have wrote may be of service to my Sisters Professors in the Art of Midwifery: and that the

the Omnipotent, Omniscient, and Omnipresent God, may grant you All Success, is the hearty and sincere Prayer, of

Your True and Faithful

Friend and Servant,

From my House in Piccadilly, over against the Right Hon the Earl of Burlington's.

Sarah Stone.

The following Letter being from a Gentleman justly celebrated in his Profession, I shall take the liberty to prefix it to this Work; and hope for the Author's excuse as well as that of the Publick, for so doing: the Motive for it being far from That of *Vanity* or *Conceit*; tho', I think, any Person may take an *honest Pride* in the Approbation of the *Worthy*.

A Copy of a Letter *from Dr.* Allen *of* Bridgewater, *to Mr.* Stone.

SIR,

I *Received Your's of the* 18th, *by which I find You and Mrs.* Stone *are removed from* Bristol, *and are settled in* London; *which I very heartily wish may be greatly to Your Advantage. Sure I am, if Knowledge and Skill in Your Professions; Honesty, Industry, and Care, will procure You Business, You will not want for a Recommendation to as many as shall be so happy as to have any Knowledge of You. You know the only Objection I had to Your leaving* Bristol *for* London, *was my Fear how You would be able to get an Acquaintance in* London, *at Your Time of Life; but I hope, That by Your own and* Mrs. Stone's *Qualifications above mentioned, You will be able to surmount that Difficulty. We have three or four Midwives in this Town at present, but they bear very poor Characters. The Place was much happier in that respect when* Mrs. Stone *began her*

her Practice here. I remember she exercis'd her Art, tho' then very young, with great Applause and Success, having been taught her Skill by the famous Mrs. Holmes *her Mother, the best Midwife that ever I knew. The great and populous Town of* Taunton *enlarged her Experience, and* Bristol *perfected and fitted her for the Metropolis,* London; *where, I hope, she will reap a very plentiful Harvest, answerable to her true Merit.*

You acquaint me that she is going to publish some Observations of her own, in the Art of Midwifery: She was so kind some Time since to shew me, in MSS. a few of those Cases; and indeed some of them were very curious and instructive. I wish it may gain her great Credit and Reputation. I shall be glad to

have

have the Pleasure of seeing it when it comes abroad, and shall truly rejoice to hear of both Your Success and Prosperity in all Your Affairs; and, according to the Compliment of the Season, wish You a happy New Year, and very many of them; who am,

Bridgwater,
Dec 25, 1736

Your Affectionate Friend

and Servant,

JOHN ALLEN.

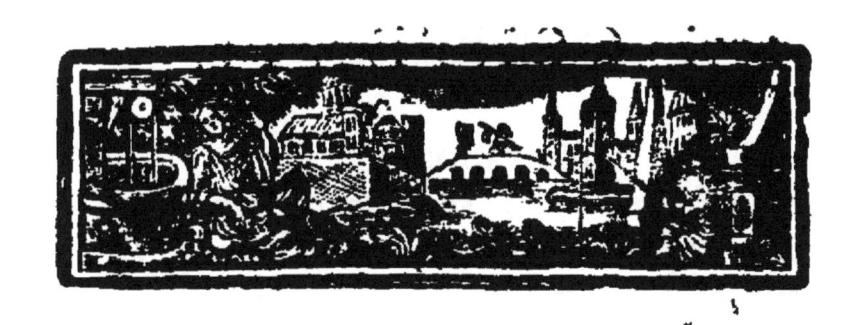

THE CONTENTS.

Observation I.
THE *Delivery of a Woman her Child being lodg'd on the Share-Bone.* Page 1

Observation II.
The Delivery of a Woman being four Days in Labour, and her Child very much Putrified. 3

Observation III.
The Delivery of a Woman in a violent Flooding, and her Child dead. 5

Observation IV.
The Delivery of a Woman, her Child being fixed on the Os Pubis, *or Share-Bone.* 8

CONTENTS.

Observation V.
The Delivery of a Woman whose Life was despaired of, her Child lying so long on the Os Pubis. Page 11

Observation VI.
The Delivery of a Woman in the uttermost Danger of Life, by the After-Burthen being left behind eight Days. 14

Observation VII.
The Delivery of two Women, their Children having a Dropsy in their Heads. 17

Observation VIII.
The Delivery of a Woman, who was likely to be ruined thro' the Ignorance of her Midwife. 23

Observation IX.
The Delivery of a Woman, the Child's Arm being without the Birth four Days. 26

Observation X.
The Delivery of a Woman, whose Child had been dead four Months, and not Putrified. 29

CONTENTS. xxvii

Obſervation XI.
The Delivery of a Woman, with the Child's Shoulder foremoſt. Page 33

Obſervation XII.
The Delivery of a Woman, her Child being dead, and much Putrified. 36

Obſervation XIII.
The Delivery of a Woman with the Child's Arm foremoſt, and much ſwelled. 39

Obſervation XIV.
The Delivery of a Woman with Twins, the one came right, and the other wrong. 44

Obſervation XV.
The Delivery of a Woman, the Child preſenting the Face foremoſt. 49

Obſervation XVI.
A Woman in the Country being delivered before I got to her Houſe, and the Child much injured. 51

CONTENTS.

Observation XVII.
Of a Woman and Child both dying, thro' the Ignorance and Weakness of her Midwife, and the Shortness of the Navel-String. Page 54

Observation XVIII.
The Delivery of a Woman, the Child having a large Tumour on the Back, and otherwise deformed. 59

Observation XIX.
A Woman in great Danger of her Life, being extreme costive, but relieved by a Glyster. 61

Observation XX.
The Delivery of a Woman who had Twins, her first Child being born the Day before. 65

Observation XXI.
The Delivery of a Woman, who was kept in hard Labour many hours by the Ignorance of her Midwife. 69

Observation XXII.
The Delivery of a Woman who had a great Flux of Blood, a Month before her Time. 73

CONTENTS.

Observation XXIII.
The Delivery of a Woman with great difficulty, her Child presenting the Arm first. Page 76

Observation XXIV.
The Delivery of a Woman, the Child having two Tumours on the Head. 80

Observation XXV.
A Woman in the Country being deliver'd before I got there, and her Child very much mangled. 82

Observation XXVI.
The Delivery of a Woman, the Child's Arm presenting first; two Midwives endeavouring to deliver, but could not. 85

Observation XXVII.
The Delivery of a Woman whose Child was dead, being very fillily managed Six Weeks before her Time. 87

Observation XXVIII.
The Delivery of a Woman in a violent Flooding, the After-Burthen presenting first. 92

Obser-

CONTENTS.

Obſervation XXIX.
The Delivery of a Woman being ſeized with the Small Pox, and brought in Labour before her Time. Page 94

Obſervation XXX.
The Delivery of a Woman, the Child's Breech preſenting firſt. 97

Obſervation XXXI
The Delivery of a Woman, the Child's Arm being out of the Birth to the Shoulder eight Days. 99

Obſervation XXXII.
The Delivery of a Woman of a Multitude of Bladders of Water. 105

Obſervation XXXIII.
The Delivery of a Woman, the Child's Knee preſenting firſt. 110

Obſervation XXXIV
A Woman being brought into great Pains and Danger before her Time by her Midwife, but went her Time out after, and both Mother and Child did well 112

CONTENTS.

Observation XXXV.
The Delivery of a Woman, the Water being broke, and kept flowing above Six Weeks before she fell in Labour, but did not go out her Time. Page 121

Observation XXXVI.
The Delivery of a Woman, who of her former Children had injured herself by too strait Lacing 126

Observation XXXVII.
The Delivery of a Woman, who had been in Labour two nights and one day, and her Pains gone, but recovered by an Anodyne. 132

Observation XXXVIII
A Woman deliver'd of her Child five days before I was sent for, and unable to make Water, relieved by a Catheter 134

Observation XXXIX
The Delivery of a Woman, whose Child's Arm presented first 137

Observation

CONTENTS.

Observation XL.
The Delivery of a Woman in a very deplorable Condition, the Child's Head lying on the Os Pubis.   Page 139

Observation XLI.
The Delivery of a Woman taken with a violent Flooding before her Time.
145

Observation XLII.
The Delivery of a Woman, with the Child's Face towards the Belly.   149

Observation XLIII.
The Delivery of a Woman, the Bottom of the Womb falling thro' its Neck.
157

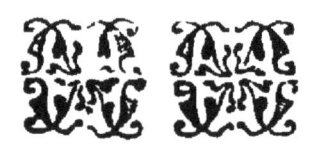

A Complete
PRACTICE
OF
MIDWIFERY.

OBSERVATION I.

The Delivery of a Woman, her Child being lodg'd on the Share-Bone.

AT *Bridgewater, Somersetshire,* 1703. I was sent for to *Huntspill,* to a Farmer's wife, who had been in Labour three days: her Pains were declining, and she reduced to the utmost degree of Weakness; not having been in Bed all that time, (which is the common, but very bad, practice of the Country Midwives.) When I came, I found her Spirits quite exhausted; and her Midwife, being also fatigued, was in a sound sleep. I laid the Woman on the Bed, and by Touching her, found the Child lay on the *Os Pubis* (or Share-bone.) The Waters being gone, made the remaining part of her Labour the more difficult: however, relieving her Child from the *Os Pubis*, which strengthen'd her Pains, I deliver'd her of a Daughter alive, and that in the space of three hours; to the grand surprize of her Midwife, when awake, who seem'd glad the Child was born alive, she believing it dead the day before.

OBSERVATION II.

The Delivery of a Woman, being four days in Labour, and her Child very much Putrified.

I WAS sent for to *Bromfield*, to a Farmer's wife, who was one of my mother's Women; and my mother being then dead about three months, she had spoke to me: but some of her friends prevailed with her to have another Midwife. The reason was, I was then thought too young, and that an elderly woman would do better. But when I came, I found the woman bolster'd upright, breatheing very short, her Nostrils working, and her Pulse very quick and irregular, as tho' Life was departing.

I ask'd the Midwife, How long she had been in that manner? she told me from Thursday, and this was on the Monday morning following. The Woman said she had not felt the Child from Friday; and, probably, it might be dead longer, by the putrefaction of the child. I could not help letting the Midwife, and women that were with her, know, That her life was in the utmost danger, proper assistance having been too long neglected; and it was my opinion, she could not long survive. They desir'd me to deliver her, which, thanks to the Omnipotent, I did, in thirty minutes, tho' with great difficulty; by reason

reason the child was so putrefied; notwithstanding which the Woman did well.

OBSERVATION III.

The Delivery of a Woman in a violent Flooding, and her Child dead.

I WAS soon after sent for to *Petherton*, two miles from *Bridgewater*, to a Taylor's wife. When I came to her she was lying on the bed speechless; for she had flooded in so violent a manner, that she never stain'd a Cloth at, or after, her Delivery. When I had stated her dangerous Case, I Touch'd her: the Secundine, I found, presented first; but Searching further, found

found the Waters not gone; wherefore having two beds in one room, I order'd the other to be ready to receive her; so breaking the Waters, the Child's head presented: but she being faint by the prodigious loss of blood, I examin'd for the Feet; which in searching for, I found the Navel-string without the least Pulsation; a plain demonstration the Child was dead. However, I found the Feet with less Difficulty than I sometimes have, and deliver'd her in less than fifteen minutes of a large boy, who, by all circumstances, had been dead about eight hours; which, no doubt, happen'd thro' her great loss of blood. As soon as I had deliver'd her of the Child and After-Birth (assisted by the Women) we laid her in the other bed. 'Twas a full hour

hour before she spoke; when she recover'd her spirits she declar'd, she remember'd not any thing of her being deliver'd. She lived and did well: for riding that way about five weeks after, I called to see her, and found her out of danger, but weak, and her Legs inclin'd to swell, which is common in such cases: but this was soon removed, by taking a few doses of proper Physick, when capable of receiving it. 'Twas 5 months before she recover'd strength enough to stir abroad; tho' had her Midwife had judgment to have deliver'd her, as soon as she fell into such Floodings, the Child's life might have been saved, and the mother preserved from extreme danger; besides the expences that such weak Lyings-in occasion, which are

are very chargeable to poor people.

OBSERVATION IV.

The Delivery of a Woman, her Child being fixed on the Os Pubis, or Share-bone.

IN a short time after I was sent for to *Bromfield*, to a Farmer's wife, who had been in Labour about eight and forty hours, her Midwife being all the time with her. She was a woman of very low spirits; her Pains were short, by reason the Child's head fix'd on the *Os Pubis* (or Share-bone.) I have observed, in all such Labours, the Pains are very short, and extreme sharp: The reason is, the

the Pains force the Child's head on the *Os Pubis*, which proves injurious both to Mother and Child. The practice of Midwives, in general, in this case, is to press hard on the back part of the body; when, indeed, they have not the least occasion to press any where; but to pass by, or thro' the *Vagina*, and gently feel for the Entrance or Mouth of the Womb; and if it be in a wrong situation, to place it right, or dilate it, as there is occasion: which I shall shew as my Observations give me leave. In this case, I examined the *Matrix*, and found the Inner Orifice lay very high to her Back, and open enough to admit of my Fore-finger, which I soon dilated to the admittance of my next finger, and with them both gently drew the *Matrix*

trix (or Womb) towards the *Os Pubis* (or Share-bone;) and as I dilated with my two fingers, at the same time, I relieved and kept back the Child's head from the *Os Pubis*. Which practice I have always found successful: for by such proceeding the Child is retarded (or kept back,) the Pains strengthened, and the Labour happily finish'd in a little time; as it hath happened to me innumerable times, in such Labours. I deliver'd this Woman in two hours, as I assured her she would be, when I first came to her: she seem'd not to credit me, but found it truth. I have attended the same Woman divers times; all her Labours are near the same, yet she and the Children do well, and hath tolerable Lyings-in.

OBSERVATION V.

The Delivery of a Woman whose Life was despaired of, her Child lying so long on the Os Pubis.

I WAS sent for to *North-curry*, to a Shoemaker's wife; I found her in a very deplorable condition, and by all her friends given to Death; for they told me, That the Shoemaker's former wife was in the very same case as this, and she died undeliver'd; and they were sure this Woman would also. The poor Woman sitting up in a chair, with the symptoms of Death in her face, and all spectators pronouncing

nouncing Death againſt her, I Touch'd her, and aſſur'd them all, that, with God's aſſiſtance, I did not doubt of delivering her in two hours; which I accordingly did: both Mother and Child did well. I have deliver'd her of ſeveral Children ſince, and ſhe is yet alive. I could not help ſmiling, to hear how the womens ſentiments alter'd; for they were poſitive in their opinions, That had I been with the firſt wife, ſhe had not died. This Woman's Caſe was much like the Woman's in the fourth Obſervation. The *Matrix* was open, and the Midwife had taken great pains to deliver this poor Woman: but inſtead of relieving the Child off the *Os Pubis*, ſhe work'd on the Back; a practice too much approv'd of by moſt authors. My principal aim in this,

this, is to inform my sisters in the Profession, That if they know how to relieve the Child from the *Os Pubis*, they need not fear; the Back-part will soon yield full fast enough for any Woman to bear: I always found it so; and have been oblig'd to support the Back-part with my hands, to prevent its being injured.

OBSERVATION VI.

The Delivery of a Woman, in the uttermost danger of Life, by the After-Burthen being left behind eight days.

I WAS sent for to a Tucker's wife in *Taunton*, in *High-Street*. She was taken with a Convulsion Fit, was two and twenty weeks gone with Child, and in the Fit the Child came from her; her Midwife, who liv'd the next door, was instantly call'd to her assistance, but could not bring the *Secundine* (or After-Birth) away. The poor Woman lay in an extreme weak condition, with continual Floodings;

ings; a Physician attended her, and order'd her Medicines to stop them. As soon as he was gone, her Midwives (for then she had three with her) consulted, and agreed to boil Herbs, and give her, to force the *Secundine* (or After-Birth) away. But soon after, she being to all human reason expiring, the Physician was sent for again, to stop her Floodings; and in that deplorable condition she lay eight days, when I was sent for. I Touch'd her, and found the Mouth of the *Matrix* open, about the breadth of a Shilling. I introduc'd my fore-finger, and then the second; and with great difficulty I brought off the After-Birth in divers pieces, very rotten and offensive. I was obliged gently to press my left hand on her Belly, to keep the *Matrix* steddy,

steddy, or else it could not have been done. The Woman recover'd, and liv'd many years, and had one Child after; contrary to the opinion of her Midwives, they thinking it impossible for her to recover. The Physician met me the next morning at her house, and gave me thanks for the service I had done his Patient. He said, 'twas always his opinion it must be brought off; but her Midwives said it could not be done. It was near five months before she recover'd strength to go abroad.

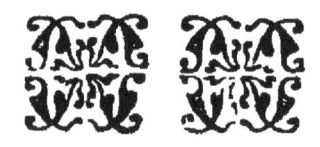

OBSERVATION VII.

The Delivery of two Women, their Children having a Dropsy in their Heads.

AT *Taunton* I attended an Inn-keeper's Wife. She was taken in Labour on a Thursday, and sent for her Midwife, who gave her hopes of a speedy Delivery. About midnight the Waters broke, and Pains a little abated, till Friday evening, and then her Pangs return'd very violent. She remain'd in that extremity till I was sent for, which was on Sunday evening: I found her more likely to die than to live, which made me unwilling

unwilling to undertake her Delivery; but she desired me, for God's sake, to do it, if she died the next moment. Her inconsoleable case oblig'd me to undertake her Delivery. In Touching her, I found the Child came with the Breech foremost, and both Feet lay across the Neck: whereupon, exerting my utmost strength, I brought the Feet to the Knees; and, with the assistance of a woman, extracted the Child to the Neck: but finding the Head stick, I search'd, and found the Head very large, and protuberant with water; the Coronal Sutures being separated at least two inches from each other, occasioned by the large quantity of water contain'd in the Child's Head. I made an Incision between the Sutures; the water flow'd freely:

ly: I then had but little difficulty to bring the Head, and soon after brought away the *Secundine* (or After-Birth.) It was very black; owing, I believe, to a Mortification she had in her Belly; of which she died the third day after Delivery. When dead, I perceived her Belly to be as green as grass, being mortified. It proceeded, as I conceive, from a great pressure often repeated, by the Women, in keeping her Belly down, according to her Midwife's directions. The reason she gave me for it was, That all the Woman's Pains, instead of Bearing down, every Pain rose up the Child, and straiten'd her Belly, round her Navel, as tho' it would have broke thro'. I laid my hand on her Belly, and it seem'd to me, that all the substance between

the Child's Head and my hand, was not thicker than fine paper. The Woman told me, That after her Waters were gone, she never had one Pain like those she used to have of her former Children; she having had seven before. I easily perceiv'd the reason, when I found the Child's Head erected as high as possible; for 'tis common for Children, whilst alive, to make the strongest efforts to be born the way the Head lies: but after this Child was dead, the largeness of the Head hindered the Pangs being successful, but, on the contrary, became very injurious. I put a Tunnel in the Child's Head, where I made the Puncture, and pour'd in five full pints of water, and judg'd it would have held half a pint more, which made the Head
prodigiously

prodigiously large, and impossible to be born of any woman in the world. And for want of this Woman's being deliver'd, when her Waters broke, she lost her life: which is very plain; for a Smith's wife, a near neighbour, and intimate acquaintance of her's, was at that time about twelve weeks gone with Child. She was often with the Woman, and saw the Child; which was a great imbecility in her, and so it is with any Woman that is pregnant, to see any thing that may affect their Infants, as this did: for two months before her Time was expired, she sent for me, and desir'd my assistance whenever her Labour came on, she telling me, she was positive her Child would be the same as her deceased friend's. She told me she was in the same way

as

as her friend; she had heard her complain often, whilst with Child: and, indeed, it proved too true. For when I was sent for to her, I found her Labour, and the Situation of the Child, and the Dropsical Head, with every particular, as the Innholder's wife. As soon as the Waters broke, I search'd for the Feet, so brought the Child's Body; but was oblig'd to make an Incision in the Head, as in the former Child. Her whole time of Delivery exceeded not an hour; the Child's Head contained near the same quantity of Water as t'other Child. She did very well, and had several Children after: which is a plain demonstration, if the other woman had been deliver'd as soon as her Waters broke, (the only time to deliver all Wrong Births) she

she might have lived; for their Labours begun equal, the Children exact alike; the bulk of the Head, and the distance of the Sutures, as tho' it had been the first Child born twice. I hope it will be a warning to all Breeding Women, that may read or know it, not to be at Difficult or Uncommon Labours.

OBSERVATION VIII.

The Delivery of a Woman, who was likely to be ruined thro' the ignorance of her Midwife.

A FEW days after I was sent for, by St. *Mary Magdelen*'s Church, to a Woman who

who had been in Labour two days and three nights. The Midwife that was with her told her friends, she believ'd she could not be Deliver'd. They hearing I was near (for I was attending on a Gentlewoman who was near her Time) sent for me. When I came, I found the Woman extremely fatigued, in a violent Transudation, that even her gown was wet with Sweat: I never saw a Woman in greater extremity. I Touch'd her, and found the Child lay right, but over the *Os Pubis*. I was surpriz'd in Touching her, to find her Fundament spread broader than the palm of my hand. I ask'd the Midwife what she had been doing: she told me that in opening the outer gate, (as she call'd it) was the way, said she, to help the inner. I was astonish'd

of MIDWIFERY. 25

nish'd at her ignorance; but have found since that it is too common a practice, even among the Men (but not the judicious) as well as Women Midwives, to work on the Back-part, which they have no business to meddle with; unless it be to support it from the injury 'tis often in danger of. I immediately endeavour'd to deliver her, by passing my two fore-fingers between the *Os Pubis* and the Child's Head. I soon reliev'd it, and in one hour and a quarter I deliver'd her of a lusty Boy. Both Mother and Child did well. 'Tis my Opinion, had I not assisted this Woman, she must soon have been ruin'd, if not lost her Life.

OBSERVATION IX.

The Delivery of a Woman, the Child's Arm being without the Birth four days.

IN *Bridgewater* I was sent for to a street below *Huntspill*, to a Farmer's wife, who had been in Labour four days. Her Midwife told me, That her Waters had broke, and the Child's Arm presented on Thursday night, and then her Pangs left her: which is very common in all Wrong Births. They sent for me on Sunday morning. I ask'd the Midwife, Why she had not help sooner? She reply'd,

She

She waited for Pains. I then inform'd her, That in all Wrong Births Pains were of no Use, but, on the contrary, pernicious. The poor Woman had been so ill used, that it was some time before I could persuade her to suffer me to Touch her, saying she chose to die, rather than go through any more Pain in that manner. I assur'd her, with the Omnipotent's leave, I would deliver her in less than half an hour. She then consented I should try. I laid her a-cross the Bed, on her Knees, with a bolster and pillow under her Stomach, that her Belly might lie hollow; which I have found, in general, to be the easiest and best way, giving liberty for turning a Child. I Touch'd her, and found the Child's Arm hal'd out, as far as the Shoulder, and

broke in two places. I slid my hand gently along the Child's Arm and Ribs, with some difficulty; so advanced further, till I found one Foot, and drew it towards me; the other soon follow'd. I wrap'd them in linnen, for the better hold, and deliver'd her, altho' the Child was much swell'd. I suppose the Infant had been dead from the Friday before. In her Delivery she never complain'd once of any Pain. I ask'd her, How she could bear the turning of her Child, and Delivery without complaining? She told me, She had endur'd a thousand times more Pain by the hands of her Midwife; and some Handy Women (as they call them) which were about her, told her, That send for whom she wou'd, she could never be deliver'd; but
they

they were soon convinced of their absurdity and brutish dealing with the poor Sufferer; for she was deliver'd, and laid in her Bed in a comfortable manner, in less than half an hour, to their great surprize. She had a good Lying-in, and was abroad in three Weeks.

OBSERVATION X.

The Delivery of a Woman, whose Child had been dead four Months, and not Putrified.

IN *Taunton*, a Smith's wife, being a Washer-woman, desired my assistance when she should want it. She told me, She had not felt the Child, since she

she quicken'd, for a month. For hanging some cloaths on a line to dry, it being out of her reach, she felt a prodigious Motion of her Child, and never felt it afterwards. Her Reckoning being almost out, she desir'd my assistance; (If she was with Child?) I told her, I did not doubt but she was; but 'twas my opinion the Child was dead from that time. She shew'd me her Breasts, which were as full of Milk, as if she had been a Nurse. She was obliged to milk them twice a day; and never milk'd less than half a pint a day, out of each at a time.

She went a Month beyond her Reckoning, and then she had several Pains. That day she sent for me in the evening: I Touch'd her, and found her Water sunk without the Neck of of the Womb: the skin that retain'd it was so very thin, that with the least touch it broke. I received some of the Water in my hand, found it very clear, and without the least putrid smell; which I wonder'd at: it being usual when a Child is dead to be offensive. Her Pains being trifling, and the *Matrix* lying high, and out of my power to reach, I order'd her to Bed, and to continue there till her Pains grew stronger: which being done, about four in the morning, she sent for me. I then found her in stronger Pains; she said they were not like the Bearing Pains she used to have with her former Children. I found the Child presented with its Breech foremost, and brought it off in a little time: but the Burden adher'd so close to the *Matrix*,

Matrix, I was obliged to peel it off, in the manner you would the rind from a young tree. And, what is worth obfervation, the Burden was at leaft two inches thick, but full as pale as the Lungs of any animal. 'Tis, therefore, plain, that altho' the Child was dead, yet that grew more than in a living Child. The Woman did exceeding well, and was capable of wafhing in three weeks after. When the Child was born, the Navel-ftring was feven times round the Neck: which palpably fhews, as the Mother was throwing a fheet over a line, the fudden jerk occafion'd the Child's being ftrangled with the Navel-ftring, the Child being whole and entire, without the leaft Putrefaction; notwithftanding it had been dead at leaft four months: an inftance

I never met with in all my Practice. I wish this may be a warning to all Women with Child, to take care not to over-reach themselves; that being often the loss of many Infants, as well as Mothers.

Observation XI.

The Delivery of a Woman with the Child's Shoulder foremost.

I WAS sent for in *Taunton*, to a Cobler's wife, who had been some time in Labour. Her Midwife told me her Child was right, which made her wonder the Child did not come forward, with so many strong Pains as she

she had for a Day and Night. I soon inform'd her 'twas the Child's Shoulder, and not the Head. I endeavour'd to place the Child right, which I did, tho' it soon return'd to the former Position. I plac'd it right three times, and still it return'd again; tho' some Authors have advised, when the Child lies not right, it must be placed so, then deliver the Woman. But I believe such Authors wrote, what they never practised; if they did, they ought to have inform'd the Readers how the Child's Head should be kept in the right Position when plac'd, and how they should procure Pains to accomplish such a Delivery: for as soon as I had placed the Child's Head right, all her Pains ceased; which is common in such Births; and obliged

obliged me to search for the Feet. I brought the Child as far as the Head; then was forced to put my two fore-fingers of my left hand into its Mouth, and gently press down the Chin to its breast with my right hand on the shoulders, and compleated the Delivery.

The Child when born had not the least appearance of life in it; but the Mother did very well soon.

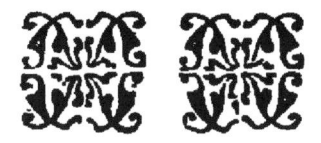

OBSERVATION XII.

The Delivery of a Woman, her Child being Dead, and much Putrified.

I WAS sent for to *Pitmister*, to a Woman who had been in Travail four days, and her Child dead the greatest part of the time; for the Skin of it flay'd off, as I deliver'd her. The Woman being very low and weak, I thought it would be least Pain to her to unbrain the Child, I being well assured it was dead, by the black offensive Water that flow'd from the *Matrix*. In such Cases, where there is a certainty of the Child's

Child's being dead, and the Head foremost, it is the easiest and quickest way of Delivery. But I think it vile practice to take such methods whilst the Child is alive, and a Woman in full strength; tho' 'tis now become too common a practice: there being many Infants born crying, with their Brains working out of their Heads. But how such Operators can clear themselves of the blood of the Infants so destroy'd, I cannot imagine; nor what their thoughts may be in such vile performances: I doubt it will give them no consoleable reflections on a dying bed. (This by way of digression.) Having no incision-knife with me, I was obliged to use a penknife. I secured the blade with a piece of rag near the point, and directed that to the

the Sutures of the Child's Head, guarding the point under the firſt joint of my fore-finger, to prevent injuring the Woman. I made a large Puncture in the Head, and then perform'd the remainder with my fingers, by taking ſeveral large pieces of the Skull and Brains; then taking hold of the back-part of the Neck, I deliver'd her in a little time. The Child was very much putrified, as was the *Secundine*, but the Woman did well. She had two Midwives with her, yet did little ſervice towards her Delivery; which they told me they wonder'd at. I made them ſenſible the difficulty was occaſioned by the Child's lying on the *Os Pubis*; for, by all circumſtances, ſhe might have been deliver'd, at leaſt, two days before, had either of of the Midwives underſtood how to have proceeded in ſuch a Labour.

OBSERVATION XIII.

The Delivery of a Woman, with the Child's Arm fore-moſt, and much ſwelled.

I WAS ſent for to a Weaver's wife in St. *James*'s Pariſh, a buſineſs ſhe was oblig'd to follow herſelf, altho' a work very injurious to Pregnant Women, eſpecially ſhort women. I have been with a great many wrong and difficult Births, I believe owing to the Woollen Trade, in which many women are obliged to be employ'd, in that town, and

and places adjacent, and no Man-midwife in the place, nor any Woman that was capable to go thro' the least difficulty; so that the whole of bad Labours lay heavy on me: which frequently happening, render'd it so fatiguing and pernicious to my health, as to oblige me to leave the place; and tho', thank God, I have recover'd since, yet I have been much concern'd to hear that many Mothers and Children have lost their lives, since my departure. One great reason of my recollecting these Observations, is, That as I cannot be serviceable in my person, I may be doubly so to those who profess or undertake the Art of Midwifery; and not to set down the least practice of any other persons, but faithfully to distribute, with the Omnipotent's tent's leave, my own performances. When I came to the aforemention'd Woman, I found the Arm hal'd out as far as the Shoulder. I ask'd, What Midwife had been with her? They said none; but I assur'd them 'twas false, and insisted on knowing who she was. Then they told me it was the Midwife that lived by; and when she heard of my being sent for, she went home: because I had been often after her bad works, and could not help condemning her for keeping Women long in hand, as she usually did, not suffering me to be sent for till the Child was dead, and the Woman in great danger. She had been with this Woman two days and one Night. I sent for her, to admonish her not to keep Women in such dangerous conditions,

tions, so long. She refusing to come, I thought it high time to deliver the Woman: I then search'd for the Feet, but found them very difficult to be come at, she being a little short Woman, and a large Child dead; the Arm and Shoulders much swell'd, which render'd her Delivery much more troublesome. I gently push'd the Child's Arm back as far as I could, which gave me a little room to slide my hand as far as the Ribs; but being seiz'd with the Cramp, oblig'd me to withdraw it: after rubbing it a little, I enter'd again, and got hold of one Foot. The Cramp seizing me a second time, I was obliged to let go my hold; but kept my hand still to ease it, and give the Woman rest: for, 'tis to be observed, when the hand is in the body,

body, and in motion, it creates great pain to the Woman. Therefore they who undertake such Deliveries, must be endow'd with great patience, justice, good judgment, and full resolution, with God's blessing, to go thro' such Deliveries. I drew the Foot towards me, which gave room to take hold of the other Foot. As the Feet advanc'd the Arm drew back. But after I had brought the Child as far as the Knees, I was obliged to have the assistance of a woman, and we both us'd all our strength to bring it to the Shoulders. I then brought down one Hand and Arm, for more room, and left the other, to prevent the *Matrix* from contracting round the Neck, which sometimes happens. I put two fingers of my left hand into the Child's mouth,

A Complete Practice

and my right hand upon its shoulders, so happily deliver'd her. I brought off the *Secundine* entirely whole.

And notwithstanding her hard Labour, she was capable of working in her Loom a fortnight after.

OBSERVATION XIV.

The Delivery of a Woman with Twins, the one came right and the other wrong.

I WAS sent for to a Woman near St. *James*'s Church; she had been in Labour from Tuesday to Friday. I found her in a low, weak condition; and, to the eye of reason, very near Death. I understood by herself

self and women, That she had been in strong Labour all that time, and quite tir'd out. Her Pulse was very low, her Breath short, her Nostrils working, so that I thought her near expireing. I ask'd her Midwife the reason, Why she did not deliver her? She told me, Because God's time was not come: (a common saying amongst illiterate and unskilful Midwives.) I told her, 'Twas my opinion, when the signs of Travail appear'd so plain, and the *Matrix* open, the Waters voided, and strong Pangs, (as had been this Woman's case, by her own confession, the Tuesday night before, and this was Friday in the afternoon) that it appear'd to me to be God's time then; and, doubtless, a Midwife's place to do her duty. The Midwife told me there was another

other reason why she had a bad time, she perceiv'd the Child had long hair. 'Tis a reason I have heard often given; but, I think, shews ignorance in abundance.

I have been frequently surprized to hear such silly reasons given, by Women practising where life is concern'd. I Touch'd the Woman, and found the Child fixed on the *Os Pubis*. I told the Midwife, I believ'd the Child had lain where it was, a considerable time. She said, Indeed she had not perceiv'd it to move (as she was pleas'd to term it) the length of a barley-corn since Tuesday night. I put the Woman on a stool, which was the way she chose; for I think it best for Midwives to advise their Women to the safest way of Delivery; which, in my opinion, none

none so good as the Bed: (and next to that the Stool) yet I don't approve of compelling Women to any particular place against their inclinations. In half an hour I releas'd the Child from the *Os Pubis*, which increas'd her Pains, so that in less than one hour I deliver'd her of a Boy. It was alive, but very weak. In searching for the *Secundine*, I met with some Membranes full of Water, which I broke, and found another Child coming with its Arm foremost. I search'd for the Feet, which I soon found, and deliver'd her of a second Son, and with small difficulty brought away the After-Births entire. I put the Woman to Bed, seemingly tolerable well for her Condition; but the next day she had a violent Fever and Purging, which

which continu'd till the fifth day, and then died.

Without dispute her Fever and Purging, proceeded from the many hot forcing things they gave her in her long and painful Travail; which is an usual, but an intolerable practice. The first Child lived two days, the second three; so that the Life of the Mother, and two Children were lost for want of judgment, and good management.

OBSERVATION XV.

The Delivery of a Woman, the Child presenting the Face foremost.

I WAS sent for to *Wilton*, to a Woman in Labour. I found her in small Pain, but the Child coming with the Face foremost, and she very low-spirited, because her Labour alter'd very much from what it used to be with her former Children. I told her, If she would keep herself on the Bed, lying on her Back till she had strong Pains, that there was no danger, and that she'd do well. She continu'd that day in small Pains

Pains till the next morning five o'clock, when I was sent for again, and about seven deliver'd her of a stout Girl, and well, except the Face, which was a little swell'd and black; a Case common when the Face presents first. In these Deliveries, if Midwives are not very careful, they may do a great deal of hurt to the Face and Eyes of the Child, as I shall shew in my next Observation, where it proved so.

OBSERVATION XVI.

A Woman in the country being deliver'd before I got to her House, and the Child much injured.

I WAS sent for to *Curry-Mallet* to a Tanner's wife, about eleven o'Clock at night, it being very bad weather, and bad roads as ever were rode, so that before I got there, the Child was born. I did not go up stairs directly to see the Mother and Child. The Women saying all was well, I thought proper to dry my cloaths, being very wet and tired, (for 'twas eight long miles.) When I had dry'd and recover'd myself, I went up stairs, and to my great surprize saw the Child with one Eye out, and the whole Face much injur'd, having no skin left on it, and the upper Lip tore quite hollow from the Jaw-bone was extremely swell'd, so that the Child could make no use of it. I put some warm water and sugar in the Child's mouth, with a small spoon, and resting it upon the Tongue, the poor Infant suck'd it down. I ask'd the Midwife, How the Child's Face came to be so miserably hurt? She told me the Mother fell down two days before she was in Travail, and, as she thought, hurt the Child, for she was sure it was born right. I told her I was sensible the Child came Head foremost, but the Face presented to the Birth; and the damage

mage the Child received was from her fingers. She could not make any defence for herself: I found her extremely ignorant.

I returned home, and sent proper dressings for the Child's Face. It did very well, and was a pretty girl, excluding the loss of her right Eye. (I saw her when she was five years of age.)

I think this Observation worth taking notice of, to caution Midwives to deal in a tender manner, when the Child presents with the Face foremost, which may be known by touching the Child. The Eyes, the Mouth, the softness of Cheeks, will sufficiently discover if the Face comes first; and then there must be waiting with patience. I have had several such Births in my time; but, I thank God, never had a Child received the least hurt, tho' a little swell'd, and blackish; which is common in those Labours.

OBSERVATION XVII.

Of a Woman and Child both dying, thro' the ignorance and weakness of her Midwife, and the shortness of the Navel-string.

I WAS sent for to a Comber's wife in *East-street*. The Woman was deliver'd of her Child about One o'clock mid-day: I was sent for at eleven at night; but it was too late; for I found the Woman dying. The relation of this misfortune,

misfortune, which I had from the Midwife and women, was this. The poor Woman was taken in Labour about twelve o'Clock, and sent for her Midwife and neighbours, who lived very near her, and by one o'Clock her Child was born. Her Midwife deliver'd her standing on her feet; (a way I cannot, in the least, approve of, tho' too commonly practis'd in the country) who being a feeble ancient woman, when the Child was born, could not bring the *Secundine* away; and the string breaking close to the head of it, occasion'd a violent Flooding, even to death: in which state I found her, quite drain'd, and past recovery. I desir'd to see the Child, and was prodigiously surprized, to see so fine a Child so unhappily and quickly lost; for

for the Bowels were in the *Omentum* or Cawl, without the Belly: and searching into the cause of such a misfortune, found it occasion'd by the shortness of the Navel-string; the Woman's standing on her feet, and the weakness of the Midwife; so that the Woman's Pains being strong and forcing, the Child was born very suddenly: and for want of the Body thereof being supported, the weight of it broke the Navel-string close to the After-Birth; and, at the same time, tore out the Child's Bowels. It was born alive, but expired in half an hour. I remember about three or four years after this misfortune happen'd, I was sent for to a gentlewoman, whom I had deliver'd of several Children. She had generally very good Times, and

I

I always deliver'd her in her Bed (which I take to be the only beſt way for Mother and Child.) When the Child was born to the pit of the Stomach, I found it would not proceed any farther, without the utmoſt ſtrength. The aforemention'd accident came in my head, and reſolving to be ſatisfy'd, I ſlid my hand to the Child's Belly, and felt the String ſtrain'd very much: I then ſlid my fingers a little farther, and ſecured the Child from danger. I kept my fingers faſt on the Navel-ſtring, and with my left hand on the back-part of the Child, accompliſh'd the Delivery. The ſhortneſs of the String occaſion'd its breaking cloſe to the *Secundine*; however, I brought the After-birth in leſs than ſeven minutes. The Mother and Child did well;

and as I have deliver'd her of several Children since, so I don't doubt but the other case, being of this nature, both Mother and Child might have been preserv'd, if the Woman had been in her Bed, and had had a Midwife of judgment and activity, which is of grand service in our Profession. I have help'd into the world many Children with short Navel-strings, but never had any misfortune attend either Mother or Child. This Gentlewoman's Child's String was not six inches long, the other about that length; the shortest I ever saw.

OBSERVATION XVIII.

The Delivery of a Woman, the Child having a large Tumour on the Back, and other ways deform'd.

I WAS sent for to a Woman of my own, which used to have very good Times, but this did not prove so. I brought the Child's Head to the Shoulders with great difficulty: and then it stuck so fast, that I was obliged to use all my strength to bring the remaining part of it; which difficulty was occasion'd by a large tumour on the Back, which reach'd from the Shoulder-blades to the Funda-

ment. In using so much strength the Tumour broke, and there was at least sixteen ounces of black matter, that resembled the Child's Excrements, if it was not the same. It appear'd when full to be quite round, and about the bigness of the crown of a child's hat; it broke in the middle of the upper part, that being the thinnest. A Surgeon was sent for to take care of it, whilst she lived; which was but eight days. I thought it a great mercy to the Infant she died. The aforesaid part on the Back being laid open, all the Backbone lay bare; and she had no Muscle in the Fundament, but a little triangular hole, as tho' made with the point of a small sword. The Excrements squeezed thro' as often as the Child's Legs were moved. The Knee-
pans

pans were under the Hams, the Feet in the place of the Ancles, and the Toes of one Foot, always lay on the Toes of the other; but it had the most beautiful Face and Hands that ever I saw an Infant have.

The Mother did well, and had Children afterwards.

OBSERVATION XIX.

A Woman in great danger of her life, being extreme costive, but relieved by a Glyster.

I WAS sent for to *Enmore*, to a Gentlewoman who was very Hysterical and Melancholy, and six Months gone with Child.
Her

Her Husband sent for a relation that lived in *Taunton,* and desir'd me to ride with her. 'Twas six long miles, eight o'Clock at night, and a very bad road; so that 'twas ten before we got there. I found her very full of Pain, and a little delirious for want of rest, not having any for a week. Her Physician had given her many medicines to prevent a Miscarriage, which could do her no service, as will appear; but what he did was occasion'd by her Midwife's informing him she was in danger of miscarrying: she told me the same, *viz.* That her Waters were broke, and she was sure she would miscarry. I desired to see some of the linnen that was wet with the Waters: They told me they were wash'd, therefore could not presently be a judge of her

her Cafe; and being a ftranger to her, fhe would not admit of my Touching her: but her hufband and relations at laft prevail'd with her, to fuffer me to fatisfy myfelf and them of her condition. It was then about three o'Clock in the morning. I told them fhe muft have a Glyfter: but fome of her friends and the Midwife were entirely againft it, thinking it needlefs; and the reafon they gave was, her being a very little eater. I told them 'twas impoffible to inform myfelf, whether fhe had any Symptoms of Mifcarriage, till the Excrements were removed; which could be no other way, with fecurity, done, than by a Glyfter. I could not perfuade them of the ufefulnefs of it, till five in the morning, when the Glyfter was given, and
fhe

she (ten minutes after) evacuated such a large quantity as surpriz'd them all; and after her second stool (for she had but two, and indeed 'twas enough) she dropt asleep, and did not wake till two of the clock in the afternoon, when she found herself easy, and quite compos'd. I then Touch'd her, but could not discover the least Symptoms of Miscarrying. She went out her Time, and did very well. She and her friends were then convinced of the advantages that did occur from that advice, I being well assured all her Pangs proceeded from the want of an Evacuation. I have observed it to be a common case among Women with Child, and always relieved them with a Glyster, and found it a means to prevent Miscarrying; altho' it is very

useful

useful to promote Delivery, when Women are at their full Time.

OBSERVATION XX.

The Delivery of a Woman who had Twins, her first Child being born the day before.

I WAS sent for to *Bishop's Lead-Yard*, to a Woman in the utmost extremity. She was taken in Labour on Friday, and on Saturday about Noon she had one Child. Her Midwife put some warm water in a close-stool, and set her on it, and desir'd her to strain with her Pains. The first Child fell into the pan of water; notwithstanding which it was alive when I came there. Her Midwife endeavouring to fetch the *Secundine*, found there was another Child, and told the Woman when the other apple was ripe, it would alfo fall. (O ignorance!) But fhe found herfelf miftaken: for on Sunday morning, her Husband came for me in a violent hurry, telling me he fear'd his Wife could not live till I got there. We rode as faft as poffible, and 'twas but five miles from *Taunton*, yet we had two meffengers fent after us for expedition, for all her Women thought her dying. When I came there I found the Child fo fixed to the *Os Pubis*, that I had an hour and half as hard work as ever I had in my life: tho' the Child was born alive, and lived till the Saturday following. The firft Child died

died the Wednesday before. I met with great difficulty in bringing the After-Births: they were very large, and extremely close join'd to the bottom of the *Matrix*. With my left hand I was oblig'd to keep her Belly down, with all my strength, whilst with my right hand I peel'd off and loosen'd the *Secundines* from the *Matrix*. My hands were seiz'd with the Cramp twice; which oblig'd me each time to hold my hand still till the Cramp was gone: which made it near twenty minutes before I could bring them both away. It was the longest time that ever I was in performing that part of my business; tho' had I been with her when the first Child was born, I should have deliver'd her of the second Child in fifteen minutes or less. For 'tis certain, if a Midwife understands her business as she ought, she might bring the second Child soon after the first: for generally in the Birth of Twins, when the first is born, the other should be brought by Art; for I never found there was any occasion either to wait for Pains, or to put a Woman to any more than ten or fifteen minutes pain, after I had deliver'd her of the first Child: especially if the first comes right, and the second wrong, as it generally proves.

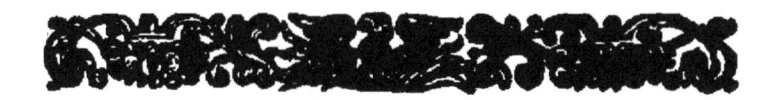

OBSERVATION XXI.

The Delivery of a Woman, who was kept in hard Labour many hours, by the ignorance of her Midwife.

I WAS sent for to *Hill-Bishops*, to a Soap-boiler's wife. Her own Midwife could not be had. Her Husband came for me; I went with him, and about a mile before we came to his house, a man met us: he was running very fast. He ask'd the man that rode before me, Whether he had seen such a Midwife? naming her name. He answer'd he had been for her, but she was eight miles off. When I came to to the Soap-boiler's house, I found the Woman in a good natural Labour: I deliver'd her in two hours: 'twas about seven o'Clock in the morning. As soon as she was deliver'd, I desir'd them to send to the afore-mention'd poor man's Wife, to know if they had got a Midwife; if not, I would go to her. They sent me word they had one, and they believ'd she would be deliver'd in a little time; but about eleven o'Clock, as I was riding home, I call'd at the house, to know if she was deliver'd: they told me no, but she would be in a quarter of an hour, so they would not give me the trouble of going in to see her. I then rode home, and about four o'Clock in the afternoon, her Husband came for me, to desire me to ride to his Wife,

for

for the women told him, they believ'd she'd never be deliver'd. I can't but say it displeas'd me, that they refus'd my seeing her, when I was so near. I went with him, and when I came, found the Woman in violent Labour. The Midwife told me the Child lay as it did, ever since seven o'clock in the morning. As soon as I Touch'd her, I was sensible of the reason of this poor Woman's being kept so long in distress. I sat down by her. She was on her Knees, one of the usual ways in the Country, but a wretched one. I found strong Pains had been so long upon her, that I could round the Head of the Child with my whole hand, when she had no Pains. The first Pain she had, after I was with her, I broke her Waters, and was forc'd to be very quick to to receive the Child; for her Pains being violent, and the Child so long confin'd by the thickness of the Skin that held the Waters, as soon as the Child had liberty, it was born in less than half a minute, which astonish'd the Midwife and Women: they would fain have prevailed on me to have told them what I did; but I chose not to inform them at that time. It is very evident, that this Woman suffer'd seven or eight hours Pain more than she need have done, had she had a Midwife of judgment in the beginning of her Travail.

I have often been sent for to the assistance of Women in the same circumstances, and have several times found them flooding. The only reason has been, for want of breaking the Waters,
the

the violent Pains opening some of the Vessels, and loosening part of the After-Birth. For 'tis an undoubted rule, If Pains do no good, they do a great deal of harm.

OBSERVATION XXII.

The Delivery of a Woman, who had a great Flux of Blood, a month before her Time.

I WAS sent for into *East-street*, to a Comber's Wife, one of my Women. When I came I found a violent Flowing of the *Menses*; and believe she lost near a gallon of Blood. She being up, I order'd her to Bed.

I ask'd her, How near she was to her Reckoning? She told me one Month. Touching her, I found little Symptoms of Labour: I told her my opinion was, she Long'd for something. She said she did not Long, but had been in pain twelve hours before her Flooding: which confirm'd my opinion touching her Longing. She still deny'd it, till I told her that both she and the Child would doubtless lose their lives, unless she speedily had what she had an Inclination for: she answer'd, What should poor people Long for? I assur'd her if 'twas any thing could be had, I would get it, let the price be what it would. She knew nothing she Long'd for, except a Peasecod, that she saw a boy hold up against the Sun: she presently after had Pains, (which

(which was the day before) Inquiring I heard of a Gentleman that had a present of some, sent him from a garden in the country, and the first that were in the town. I got some of them for her: as soon as she had eaten them her *Menses* ceas'd. She went the Time of her Reckoning, and had a good Labour. I deliver'd her of a Son: the Child and Mother both did well. Such things as these frequently happen.

Therefore have reason to believe that Forc'd Deliveries in these Cases, have destroyed many Lives. I could give various Instances of this kind in my practice, but chuse only this by way of caution, because Women are very apt to conceal their Longings, which makes them often very great sufferers thereby.

OBSERVATION XXIII.

The Delivery of a Woman, with great difficulty, her Child presenting the Arm first.

I WAS sent for to a School-Mistress: when I came, I found her Pains small, her Waters broke four days before: she was very ill, and had a Fever. I Touch'd her, and found the Child lay a-cross. One Arm and the Ribs presenting first, the Waters being past, and her Body hot and dry, I apprehended 'twould be a difficult Labour; and so it proved: for as I slid my fingers along the Ribs, to search for

for the Feet, my Hand and Arm was so seized with the Cramp, as obliged me to withdraw my Hand for fifteen minutes. I attempted again, but without success. I was very uneasy, knowing such attempts put the Woman to fresh Pain. In short, I was forced to rest till my Arm was better, when I made another attempt, and, with God's leave, perform'd the Delivery, without withdrawing my Hand any more, although my Hand was several times numbed, before I could reach the Feet: but as I advanced I found the Child alive, and suck'd my finger in the Womb, which concern'd me; fearing it impossible for the poor Infant to be born alive, because of the circumstances already given; the Mother's weakness, and the Child's largeness. But recovering

recovering my thoughts, I resolved to do my duty for the poor Woman's sake, and leave the event to the Omniscient God. I was obliged to be exceeding careful and slow, yet resolved with all my strength, and a full resolution, to accomplish what I was about. When I had hold of one Foot, I found it hard work to hold it, and draw it towards me, by reason I could hold it but with my two fore-fingers at first. However, I kept my hold, and in a small time brought the Feet out of the *Uterus* (or Womb.) I brought also the Legs out to the Knees; then I wrapt them in a linnen cloth, and gave them to two strong Women, and desir'd them to draw in a strait line, whilst I took care of the Woman's body,

to

to prevent any injury, and secure the Child that it might be brought off whole; which, thro' mercy I compleated. The *Secundine* ftuck clofer to the *Matrix* than is common in thefe Cafes; which, I believe, was owing to the drynefs of the Womb from her Fever. The Child had not the leaft appearance of life, and 'twas impoffible it fhould: this Delivery being at leaft an hour and half's hard work, which feldom happens: for in common wrong Births it is very rarely more than half an hour, and often not fifteen minutes. I don't remember above four fuch terrible Labours, in all my practice. The Woman did well. I have fet this Obfervation down as plain as poffible, to encourage Midwives, that they may with juftice and fafety go thro' the

moft

most difficult part of their work, as well as that which is easy. I could not turn in my bed, without help, for two or three days after, nor lift my Arm to my Head for near a week; and forced to bathe my Arm with Spirit of Wine several times a day.

OBSERVATION XXIV.

The Delivery of a Woman, the Child having two Tumours on the Head.

I WAS with a Comber's wife, a near neighbour to the Woman mention'd in my last Observation: she had been in Labour, and her Midwife with her several days. I ask'd the Midwife

wife the reason why she did not deliver her. She could give me no account, whether the Child was right or wrong; but Touching her, I found the Shoulder-blade presented first. I advanc'd farther in search of the Feet, and found the Child's Navel-string without the least Pulsation, which satisfy'd me 'twas dead. I found the Feet, and drew them towards me, so compleated the Delivery in less than half an hour. Viewing the Child, I saw on the back part of the Head two large Tumours, one above the other, as if the Water contain'd in the under Tumour, did, when full, ascend to the upper one, which reached to the Crown of the Head. The biggest was as large as a Goose's egg, and the other about half that size. I open'd them both; 'twas

'twas only clear Water that issued out of them: it lay between the hairy Scalp and the Skull. The Woman did well; but had a Fever for five days; which I imputed to some strong waters given her for her Pains, as they said; which I think a pernicious Custom.

OBSERVATION XXV.

A Woman in the country being deliver'd before I got there, her Child being very much mangled.

I WAS sent for to *Hatch*, to a Farmer's wife, but before I could get there a Midwife had deliver'd her: she was in a very low

low condition, more likely to die than to live. The Child was sew'd up in a piece of Flannel, and cover'd with Flowers in order for its Burial. I desir'd to see the Child, but the Midwife refus'd for some time. I insisted on its being undress'd, which was accordingly done. When I saw the Infant, I was much surprized; for the left Arm was tore off, in a most indecent manner. I ask'd the Midwife, If she was sure the Child was dead before she proceeded in so rash a manner? She told me she did not know but it was: for the Arm had been in the world above thirty hours. I never saw a Child so mangled in my life. The Midwife seem'd to have more Courage than Judgment. The Woman likewise received great hurt;

hurt; but taking my advice she recover'd. I heard from her every other day, till she was out of danger. I could not constantly attend her, it being eleven miles from me, and very bad roads.

I should not have mention'd this error of the Midwife's, had it not been to caution others against attempting such Deliveries without knowledge. I told her, if she had proceeded in a regular manner, as soon as her Waters broke, to have search'd for the Feet, she might have turn'd it, and deliver'd the Woman, without mangling the Child, or injuring the Mother. She acknowledg'd what I said was very just; and that she would not proceed so rashly for the future.

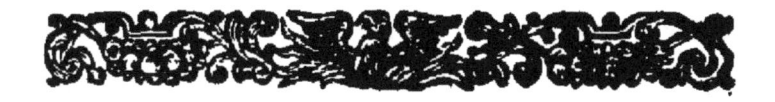

OBSERVATION XXVI.

The Delivery of a Woman, the Child's Arm presenting first; two Midwives endeavouring to deliver, but could not.

I WAS sent for to a Comber's Wife, who had two Midwives with her for a Day and a Night, endeavouring to turn the Child; but finding it not in their power, they then desir'd my assistance. I found the Woman leaning forward on the back of a chair, and both the Midwives at hard labour; but the poor Woman at much harder. I laid her on the bed, on her left side, and

and search'd for the Feet, which I easily found. I turn'd the Child, and deliver'd her with a great deal of ease in less than ten minutes. For the Midwives endeavouring to return the Child's Arm (as they told me they had done several times, but it would not remain in the Body) had made such way, that occasioned the Delivery to be easy to me, altho' the Woman was a great Sufferer by such management. I never found any occasion in those Births to return the Arm; I always found liberty enough, with gentle proceeding and strength, to pass by the Arm, and come at the Feet, which always succeeded well. The Child had been dead some time, but the Mother recover'd.

OBSERVATION XXVII.

The Delivery of a Woman whose Child was dead, being very sillily manag'd Six Weeks before her Time.

IN *Paul's Street*, I was sent for to a Woman that thought herself in Labour; but I told her the Pain she had was the Cholick. I order'd her something to take, and advis'd her to go to bed. I went home, it being after ten at night. I sent the next morning to know how she did her mother sent me word she had a good night, and was then asleep.

I was sent for to a Gentlewoman in the Country on a Miscarriage

carriage that morning, where I remain'd that day. In the afternoon the Woman was seiz'd with the Cholick again: her Husband came for me; but I being with the Gentlewoman, they got another Midwife. I came home about six in the evening, and went to see how the Woman did. Her Husband met me at the door, and told me that not being at home, he had got another Midwife; and that his Wife was like to be deliver'd in a little time: I said I was sure 'twas impossible. I went home without seeing the Woman, but sent three times that night, to know how she was; the constant answer was, she was on the pinch of Delivery. I heard nothing of her for three days after; and then I was told the poor Woman was not deliver'd. The news did not surprize me, I being well assured her Time was not expired; nor her Pains, when I was with her, the least tending to Labour. I immediately went to see her, and found her in a very low condition; her Midwife and Women with her. They told me they had been with her all that time: Her Eyes were swell'd with weeping; her Midwife having told her, she thought she could never be deliver'd. I ask'd the reason, Why she kept the Woman so long in hand? She said, Because God's time was not come: I told her, I then thought she had no business with her. The reason she gave for trying to deliver her, was because she had Pains. I Touch'd the Woman, but found not the least Symptoms of Labour, only the

Birth extended and swell'd, thro' the ill usage and ignorance of her Midwife. I order'd her to be put to bed, and gave her things to ease her Pains, which had been much increas'd by ill management. I bid them keep her in bed three or four days, till all her Pains were gone. I order'd Fomentations for the parts swell'd. She went Six Weeks after this, in which time I often saw her: she continually complain'd of a constant Motion of the Child, which made her so weak for want of rest, that she was incapable of doing any business. At the Six Weeks end she sent for me, about eight of the clock at night, and told me she had Pains; but had not felt her Child for two days. I Touch'd her, and told her 'twou'd be her Labour; but I could

could be no ways serviceable to her till morning. I bid her keep in her bed till her Pains came stronger, which she accordingly did; and about nine the next morning she sent for me again. About eleven o'clock, I deliver'd her of a Boy, which, I believe, had been dead the whole time that she had not felt it. It was like a Skeleton, cover'd with a beautiful white Skin; but the Bones and Ribs plainly appear'd thro' the Skin. It was exceeding tall. I doubt not but the Child's being disturb'd before its Time, was the Cause of its continual Stirring; and, consequently, of its extreme Thinness and Death.

This Observation I have set down to caution those professing the Art of Midwifery, to be well assur'd of a True Labour, before they begin their Work.

OBSERVATION XXVIII.

The Delivery of a Woman, in a violent Flooding, the After-Burthen presenting first.

I WAS sent for into the Country, about seven miles distant from my house, to a Butcher's Wife. Her Husband told me, the Women order'd him to make all possible haste, for they fear'd she would die before I got there. I found her very low and weak; for she had had a continual Flowing of the *Menses* for a Fortnight, and then flooded ed so violently, that she was given over. She had two Midwives with her: they said that the Woman told them, she was Six Months gone with Child; but they could not believe it; for by searching her they could not perceive any Child. I then thought it highly necessary to inform myself of the reasons of her violent Flooding; and Touching her found a great deal of Coagulated Blood, which I brought off, and then perceived the After-Birth to present first: I got that immediately; and then brought off the Child 'Twas a fine Boy, and lived about half an hour. By its Largeness, I believe, she was near Seven Months gone. The Woman lived and did well, but it was some Time before she recover'd her strength.

O b-

OBSERVATION XXIX.

The Delivery of a Woman being seized with the Small Pox, and brought in Labour before her Time.

I WAS sent for to *North Curry*, to a Woman that had been in Labour two days and one night; but in no more likelihood of being deliver'd, than when her Midwife was first with her, as she told me; altho' she had been in strong Pains ever since, and in a high Fever. I Touch'd her, and found it not a natural Labour: but being kept so long in hand endeavouring to procure a Delivery, the Waters

Waters were gone, and part of the Child's Head bare. The Child being dead, I thought it proper to use my utmost endeavour to deliver her, which I accordingly did, and in a short time brought off the *Secundine*. It was very whole and sound; but after her Delivery she complain'd of a violent Pain in her Back, and said she was almost as bad now as when in Labour. I consider'd what might be the reason of her Complaint, knowing she was safely deliver'd; I was satisfied her Pangs could not proceed from her Labour. I ask'd her, If she had ever had the Small Pox? She told me No; and that she had been six miles from home, and in the house where she lay there was a person in the Small Pox, who surpriz'd her very much: 'twas three days

days before she fell ill: she said she had Six Weeks longer to Reckon. I order'd her Husband to send for a Physician, for by her violent Fever, and Lightheadedness, she was in great danger of Life; and so it proved: for she did not live above eight and forty hours, but died delirious. Her Daughter-in-law came to me after she was bury'd, and told me she was prodigiously full of the Small Pox and Purples; and that it was the opinion of the Physician, had they sent for him at first, when she sent for the Midwife, both she and the Child might have been preserved: for her Midwife, whilst with her, had given her strong Waters and her Husband's Water with the juice of Leeks, and other things of the same nature, keeping her out of her bed; all

all which management increas'd her Fever, and forc'd her Labour; tho' all her Pains at first were only Symptoms of the Small Pox.

OBSERVATION XXX.

The Delivery of a Woman, the Child's Breech presenting first.

I WAS sent for to *Creech*, to a Gentlewoman that I usually deliver'd. She told me she had Pains, but believed she should die. She was always a timorous, fearful Woman, but now more so than formerly. I found her Child was wrong, and was some time before I could perswade her to go to bed: I prevail'd prevail'd with her at last, and got her in bed without breaking her Waters, which answer'd my ends. I laid her on her left side, and the first and second Pains she had, after she was in bed, I dilated the *Matrix*, which sunk the Waters very low and large; in her third Pain I broke the Waters, and slipt my finger in the Bending of the Child's Thigh, for it came Breech foremost, and so deliver'd her in less than three minutes. But notwithstanding she had so quick a Delivery, and good Lying-in, and that both Mother and Child did well; yet some of her Women said they should not like a Midwife to bring a Child so quick; but they lik'd a Midwife to stay and wait till Pains brought the Child: as will appear in the following Observation,

tion, where they kept the Woman a long time in suspence, without sending for me, for fear I should deliver her too soon.

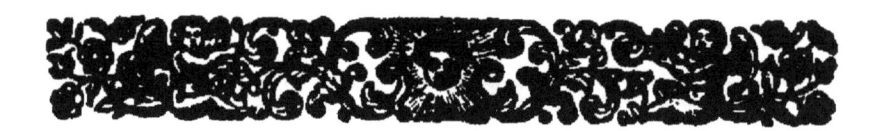

OBSERVATION XXXI.

The Delivery of a Woman, the Child's Arm being out of the Birth to the Shoulder eight days.

SOME Time after I was sent for, in the Parish of *Creech*, to a Woman who had been in Labour nine days. Her Husband came for me on a Saturday in the Afternoon, and the Child's Arm had been out of the Birth to the Shoulder the Saturday before; which was eight whole days,

days, and, by circumstances, near as long dead. Her Midwife told me her Pangs came on strong the Friday sennight before in the Evening, and early on Saturday Morning her Waters broke, and then the Child's Arm came forth from the Womb, and her Pains immediately went off. She had had none since that time till now, and she believ'd the Child dead from the Saturday Noon; for whilst it was living it often clasp'd its hand round her finger, but had long ceased to do so. She had look'd on the Hand and Arm of the Child, and found it black, and much swell'd; which is common as soon as a Child is dead: the Blood always settling in that manner. Her information seem'd to be very right; for had it been dead and bury'd

three

three months, I think it could not have been more putrified nor offensive. I instantly endeavour'd to deliver the Woman, by searching for the Feet, but her Pains were so violent, as to force the Child so strong against my hand, that my attempts proved all in vain. I then consider'd I should want an Incision-knife, to take off the Arm at the Shoulder, (a thing I never had need to attempt before.) But having neither Incision-knife, nor Pen-knife, I took hold of the Arm, to try if I could twist it off, and with a very small pull it dropp'd from the Body. I then proceeded to search for the Feet, which I soon found. The first Foot I got hold of I drew towards me, but it immediately separated from the Knee: I laid it it down, and search'd for the other, and that came off likewise: then I took hold of one Thigh, and brought that to the Birth; and with my other hand got hold of t'other Thigh, and brought both together in a strait line. The Woman's endeavours with her Pains very much assisted me to bring off the remaining part of the putrid Body, which I brought off together very soon, and rescu'd the poor Woman from the Jaws of Death. For the violence of her Pains had distracted her so, that she often begg'd the Women to kill her. Had she not been deliver'd soon she must have died; for when I came there, I beheld her an object in such violent bearing Pains, I believe the strongest that ever were seen or felt. Which confirm'd me in my opinion,

opinion, That Women never die undeliver'd for want of Pains. For had her Child been right, it would have been born with two or three such Pains, without a Midwife; but as it lay wrong, it was impossible to be born by the strength of ten, without judgment.

I compleated the Delivery of the Child and After-Birth, within three quarters of an hour. The Woman recover'd, and did well, although her Blood was as green as the top of a standing pond; which was occasion'd by her Child's being so long dead, and giving her such quantities of strong Waters, and her Husband's Water with the Juice of Leeks; which is a notable Prescription among Country Midwives, but a horrid Medicine, and as often mischievous as prescrib'd.

scrib'd. The Midwife told me, The reason of giving these hot things was to promote her Pangs: I told her, I never gave one thing to increase Pains in all my Practice. For Pains were no longer useful in Wrong Births, than till the Waters broke. And if she would know whether a Child lies Right or Wrong, before the Waters break, she must search very gently between the intervals of her Pains; for then the Waters slacken, and 'tis easily discover'd what part of the Child presents first. If 'tis Wrong, a Midwife ought to be in readiness, and endow'd with judgment, to Deliver her Woman; which may be done in fifteen or twenty minutes.

OBSERVATION XXXII.

The Delivery of a Woman of a Multitude of Bladders of Water.

I WAS sent for to a Sergemaker's Wife; She told me she was in the Seventh Month of her Pregnancy. She was taken with a violent Flowing of the *Menses*. She sent for her Midwife; but she doing nothing for her, she sent for a Physician: he gave her medicines that retarded them for a time. In about a fortnight they return'd again, and so continu'd every twelve or fourteen days, till her Life was despair'd of. She told

told me she had commonly small Pains, before the return of her Flooding. I told her 'twas my opinion, That at the return of those Pains, what was in the *Matrix* must be brought off. I also assur'd her, I did not think it was a Child: she said she was sure it was, tho' it might be weak, for she felt it. I took my leave of her for that time: about eight days after she sent for me in great haste, her Pains being return'd; but by the time I got there her Pains were almost gone. On examining, I found the entrance of the *Matrix* open enough to admit the top of my fore-finger, and by force I advanc'd my second finger. I was obliged to press my left hand strenuously on her Belly, to keep the *Uterus* steddy, and with my two fingers I brought off
a

a great quantity of Bladders of Water; the largeſt about the ſize of a Pigeon's Egg, and ſome as minute as a ſmall Pin's-head. I brought off near twenty parcels that hung together, with a putrified Fleſh. I put it in a large baſon, for her Phyſician to ſee. It was his opinion 'twas a Falſe Conception: but 'tis my opinion 'twas a True Conception for the firſt ten Weeks, and at that time ſhe loſt the Child; the After-Birth remaining behind, grew to that Subſtance. For I have often obſerv'd the *Secundine*, in many Miſcarriages about eight or ten Weeks gone, to have been no other than a ſpungy Subſtance, full of ſmall Bladders of Water, the bigneſs of Pepper-Corns, and ſome much ſmaller, and the *Fœtus* ſeated in the middle of a Bladder of Water, as large as a Hazel-nut. This Woman miscarried six times before she had a living Child: then she had a Son, and a good time. The next time of being Pregnant she miscarried about the usual time; and never miscarried without imminent danger of Life, thro' a great loss of Blood. I have thought her dead when I have enter'd the room, but as soon as I Touch'd her (I thank the Omnipotent for that knowledge) I never failed stopping her Flooding. I brought off all her Conception, before I could venture to leave her. When Pregnant again, (which was the second time of conceiving after her Son) it proved to be of the same nature as the former, consisting of Bladders of Water, to the quantity of two quarts. She did not

not exceed twenty two Weeks, before she was in the same dangerous condition; when her Pains being tolerable strong, I brought it off in fourteen minutes: and yet, after this, she went her Time with a Daughter, and I left her well, with the Child sucking at her Breast. In six or seven Months after I left *Taunton*, which was the place of her residence, I was inform'd by her friends, that she had wean'd that Child, and was Breeding again. I was concern'd to hear it, but wish'd she might go her Time and do well; but was inform'd to the contrary in less than three Months after, and that she was dead, and ended Life with a violent Flooding, the Conception not being brought off.

OBSERVATION XXXIII.

The Delivery of a Woman the Child's Knee presenting first.

I WAS sent for to a Weaver's Wife in *East-street*. She had had several Children, but all dead born by the misfortune of their lying wrong. This was the first time I was with her. I found the Child Wrong, and could not instantly discover what Part presented first; her Pains following so fast, that they would not give the Waters time to slacken. As soon as her Waters broke, I found it was the Knee presented. I then endeavour'd deavour'd to slide my Finger in the Bending of the Knee, which I brought forward: I got the other, but with some strength, which forced the Woman's Pains. I soon deliver'd her of a Son alive and well. I always found when a Child comes that way, it may be born with little difficulty, without searching for the Feet (which some Authors direct to) and that without any hurt to Mother or Child; having deliver'd many Women of such Births. The greatest difficulty I ever found, was to be very quick in bringing the Child to the Birth, whilst the Pains were strong, just on the breaking of the Waters: and not to be too busy in such Labours, till there is a sufficient prospect; then the Work will be soon finish'd with credit.

OBSERVATION XXXIV.

A Woman being brought into great Pains and Danger before her Time by her Midwife, but went her Time out after, and both Mother and Child did well.

I WAS sent for to a Shepherd's Wife at *King's-Clift.* Her Husband told me she had been in Labour from Saturday, and he came for me Monday in the Afternoon. I found the Woman much fatigu'd, having had a great many small Pains, but found they were not Labour Pangs; although her Midwife often call'd for the Receiver

to

to take the Child, on Sunday night. When I came and heard what had been done, I told her I was certain the Symptoms of Labour the Woman had upon her, were the effect of her too frequently Touching her. For I found the *Uterus* open the breadth of a Crown-Piece. I then ask'd the Woman if her Reckoning was out? She told me 'twas not full nine Months since she had her first Child, and she went but eight Months with it; which made her Midwife and Women to believe she would go no longer with this. I told them, in short, 'twas not her Labour, and if she would follow my directions, I did not question but she would go her full Time. They said they would not believe it: but the Woman herself said, She would take my advice.

vice. I order'd Nurse to put her to bed, and keep her there at least two Days; and told her what Fomentation to make, and to use it warm three times a Day, till all her Disorders were taken off, which the Midwife had brought on her, by her too busy Touching. I charg'd the Woman, when she was taken in True Labour (which I inform'd her how to know) That she should keep her bed, and not rise as soon as she felt her first Pangs: a way common in the country; nor to send for her Midwife too soon. She told me she hoped I would come to her: I answer'd, I was sensible her Time would be so quick, that it would be in vain to send for me; neither would she have any occasion: for a good Motherly Woman might be able to deliver

deliver her; and I am sure, many Women would fare much better, if they committed themselves to God and Nature, than to employ ignorant Midwives. I went home, and sent her proper Medicines to ease her Pain, and the Saturday following, which was our market-day, her Husband came to me, and told me his Wife was brave and well; he hoped she would go her Time out, and have a live Child; the first being born dead. I told him I did not question it.

That day three Weeks he came to my house again, and told me his Wife was deliver'd of a Daughter, about two of the clock that morning. And as I observed to her it happen'd; for before the first neighbour could get to his house, the Child

Child was born. His Wife and Child were both well. In six Weeks after she came to see me, and return me thanks for my advice: and told me she was certain her first Child would have been born alive, had she sent for me, and herself freed from a great deal of misery, that she went through; she also affirm'd she was better, and stronger in one Week, than she was of the first Child in three Months.

OBSERVATION XXXV.

The Delivery of a Woman, the Water being broke, and kept flowing above six weeks before she fell in Labour, but did not go out her time.

I WAS sent for to a Gentlewoman, that I had deliver'd of all her Children, she having had several before this. I found her in a great surprize; she told me she thought herself five months gone with Child, but, as she sat at Dinner, her Water broke, and a large quantity came off; it still continued, yet she declared she had not the

least

least pain. I told her there was no Danger in her Case, if she would take my advice, To keep herself very quiet. She asked me if I thought she should go her Time? I answered, I much question'd it; but keeping herself quiet, was the only thing I could advise, to prevent Miscarrying. She continued six weeks and four days, her Waters constantly running all that time: She was then taken with small Pains, and sent for me; I told her it would prove her Labour, though not so quick as her other Labours used to be, when at her full time. She was in Bed when I went to her, it being early in the morning; I desired she would keep herself there, which she did, and about three hours after, her Pains came stronger, that in a little time I delivered

delivered her of a Son, alive, and in good case, considering the time she went with it, which was six months fourteen days. There did not appear the least Disorder in the Child, from her Waters being broke so long before its time. The Child being born so long before the usual time, was the occasion of its death, for he lived but a few hours; and the reason of her Travail being more lingering than when at her full time, was from the Unnaturalness of her Labour, which I have observed is seldom otherwise in cases where Women come before their time. I should not have mentioned this, (because I have had many such Births in my Practice) were it not that many Women are apt to be much discouraged when such Circumstances

stances happen to them. About five Years ago, one of my Women sent for me, and, when I came, told me she was much surprized and frighted, for her Waters were broke, and that without Pain: She had a month longer to reckon, and fear'd it was a token of her death, because her Children always followed her Waters; I gave her for reason of this Alteration, That it often happen'd, from the thinness of the Membranes, and the weight of the Waters, and told her it was my opinion she would go her time, as many had to my knowledge. I gave her many instances of this nature. She went a month longer, which completed her Reckoning; but she fatigued me daily, sending for me, and telling me that one Friend and another strove

strove to persuade her that they were certain she must be in great danger, and asked why she did not send for a Man, and be delivered? I told her, she might use her pleasure, for my part, I apprehended no Danger attending her, and that I never had one Woman do amiss in my Life in her Case, and did not doubt her doing well, when her time was expired. And so she did, and had the quickest and best time that ever she had before or since.

The best Advice I can give, and what I always found successful, whenever a Woman's Water breaks (let the time be long or short, before their Reckonings are expired) is, to keep themselves as Quiet as possible, and take care they get no Cold, and then to wait with Patience,

Patience, and not to lay any Stress on Nature, nor in the least to use any Art, or Endeavours to promote a Delivery.

OBSERVATION XXXVI.

The Delivery of a Woman who of her former Children had injured herself by too Strait Lacing.

A Farmer's Wife that lived two Miles in the Country, came to speak with me, and told me, she had four months to reckon, tho', by her Bigness, I thought she could not have one; but she told me, she was sure it was so. I then told her, I fear'd she

she laced very tight; she said it was what she was advised to by her Midwife, and Acquaintance in the Country. I answer'd, it was a great Error, and that she ought to give herself all the Liberty possible; she seemed very much rejoiced, for she said she was usually sick, and fainted three or four times a day. She begg'd I'd let her Husband hear my opinion; for of her two former Children she was in Labour a week each Child, and both dead born, which the Women told her Husband was owing to her not lacing straight enough. Her Husband returning to my house in about half an hour, I told him the Advice I had been giving his Wife, but that she did not incline to follow it without his approbation. He immediately acquiesced to what

what I said, and desiring her to lace moderately the rest of the time, he declared 'twas a great concern to him to see her in those fainting Fits; but that his greatest desire being to have a Child alive, made him persuade her to bear her lacing. I cannot imagine what Advantage any Woman can receive from severe lacing; but, on the contrary, have known it very injurious, especially to such short Women as this was; for the *Pelvis* in such being much shorter, of consequence must be less than in tall Women; and were they to lace below the *Os Pubis*, they could not walk. So that all the room above the Share bone being little enough to contain a Child, certainly such people as do advise straight lacing, never saw a Woman open'd, open'd, undeliver'd; if they had, they could not be of that Opinion, but advise them rather to wear no stays; for to see in what little room the Bowels are confined, and especially when the Child is very large, it is astonishing that Women and Children do well; what can be said for it is, the Omniscient that form'd us in the Womb, hath ordered it so.

According to the Woman's Reckoning, about four months after, I was sent for about ten at Night, and finding her up, order'd her to bed; she ask'd me, What she should do there, for she never went to bed when in labour in her life? However, she agreed to be ruled by me, and went to bed. About eleven o'clock, I sat down by her, and found my assisting her, (in put-
ing

ing my two fingers just within the entrance of the *Uterus*) strengthened her Pains, and with every Pain brought it forward to the *Os Pubis*. Her Child proceeded very fast, for by this method I am always capable of strengthening and lengthening a Woman's Pains, if in true Labour. About twelve of the clock, she began to be very impatient, and desir'd to rise, but was no sooner up, than she begg'd to go to bed again. I told her, if she would go to bed again, there she must be delivered; and, accordingly, about one o'clock I laid her in a proper posture for that purpose, and, (by the before-mentioned method of bringing the mouth of the *Matrix*, above the *Os Pubis*, with every Pain, till the Child's head was

was quite clear from it) I delivered her, in about an hour, of a Son, a very stout Child, and alive.

I have endeavoured to be very plain in this Observation, that if the Readers professing the Art of Midwifery have the least genius, they may soon arrive to be great proficients in this Art.

OBSERVATION XXXVII.

The Delivery of a Woman who had been in Labour two Nights and one Day, and her Pains gone, but recover'd by an Anodyne.

I WAS sent for to a *Comber's* Wife, by *East Gate*. I found she had been in Labour two nights and one day. Her Midwife told me her Pains were gone, and altho' she had given her their usual Prescriptions, a large quantity of Dr. *Stevens*'s Water, and her Husband's Water, with the juice of Leeks, (often mentioned) they did not strengthen her Pains. I found her

her Pangs small, and a great distance between them; notwithstanding I could round the Head of the Child to the Ears. I order'd her Nurse to warm the bed hot, it being cold weather, and, as soon as she was in bed, gave her an *Anodyne*, (which I have always found successful in lingering Labours, to remove unprofitable Pains, and facilitate the Birth in true Labours) which, according to my expectation, succeeded; she soon fell asleep, and continued sleeping and dosing for six hours; soon after she wak'd, her Pains came on stronger; I was sent for again, and found her Pains, with my assistance, (as in the former Obsevation,) answered the desired Ends of a speedy Delivery: but her Child was dead; and, its skin being full of blisters of water, appeared to have been dead some time. However, the Woman did well, notwithstanding the length of her Labour.

Observation XXXVIII.

A Woman delivered of her Child five Days before I was sent for, and unable to make Water, relieved by a Catheter.

I WAS sent for to *East-Street*, to a Gentlewoman who had been delivered five Days, and made no Water in all that time, but brought up most she took, and was in continual Pain. She was extremely swelled, and her Belly

Belly much bigger than it was before her Delivery. I was obliged to make use of a *Catheter*, and immediately drew off more than a gallon of water, which gave her great ease for the present. She had a Physician from the second day; he order'd her Fomentations to her Belly three times a day. I was forc'd the next day to draw off her water again. When her Physician ask'd me my opinion, what was the matter with her? I told him I thought an Inflammation of the Womb: He said, that was very contrary to what her Midwife told him. I gave him for reason, that in Touching her, I found the Womb exceedingly swelled, and very hard. I continued to draw off her Water once a day, for eight days. Her Vomiting still continued,

tinued, with a violent Fever, and her Cleanfings quite ftop'd; and altho' her Phyfician, (a Gentleman of Eudition and Judgment) ordered her a great many proper medicines for that cafe; yet fhe continued a fortnight more like to die than to live; but the fixteenth day after her Delivery, fhe was taken with a violent Purging, and had near forty ftools in twenty-fix hours, and, though what fhe voided was very black, and infupportably offenfive, yet, by the care of her Phyfician, fhe recovered, and did well.

OBSERVATION XXXIX.

The Delivery of a Woman whose Child's Arm presented first.

I WAS sent for to a *Comber's* Wife in St. *James's* Parish, about eight of the Clock at night, but, being very ill of the Cholick, could not go. They told me she had a Midwife with her, but she could not deliver her; and about twelve o'clock I was called again; but continuing very ill, they sent for another Midwife. About five of the clock in the morning, they sent again, and told me the Woman would die, if I did

I did not go to her assistance, for neither of her Midwives could deliver her. This oblig'd me to rise and go with them, altho' I was so ill as to be forced to hold by the Woman's Husband and another. When I got there, I found the Child's Arm out of the Birth; I immediately searched for the Feet, which I soon found, and in a little time completed the Delivery. I was led home, and in my bed before the clock struck six. This fixed my Resolution of leaving *Taunton*, for the Country Business was too hard for me; having no conveniency in any Illness, but obliged to go on horseback, or foot, which had so impaired my health, that, notwithstanding it is sixteen years since I left it, I enjoy more health and strength, than

I did

I did at that time; for I brought at least three hundred Children a year into the World, for many years before I left the town. I could enumerate vast numbers of these *Observations*, but have set down only a few, which, I hope, will prove beneficial to my sex in general, when in my grave.

OBSERVATION XL.

The Delivery of a Woman in a very deplorable Condition, the Child's Head lying on the Os Pubis.

I WAS sent for to *Paul's Sreet*, to a Gentlewoman, her own Midwife being from home. She said

said she usually had very good Times, but was more uneasy the last three months of her time, with this Child, than ever she was before, altho' this was her eighth child. She said her Child lay exceeding forward, which occasioned her a great deal of Pain, in the lower Part of her Belly and Groin. When I Touch'd her, I soon let her know the reason of her Pain; the Child was a little lodged on the *Os Pubis*, which caused a sharper Travail than any she had before, although I delivered her in the space of two hours. Her Husband's relations persuaded her it was owing to the Change of Midwives; however, she was willing to have me at her next Delivery, but they would not consent to it; so she had her own Midwife again, and had

had as good a time as ever; which confirmed her relations in their opinion, that the fault was in the Midwife. But being with Child again, she very often complained that she was in the same manner, and as uneasy as she was of the Child that I delivered her of. When her time was expired, and she was in Labour, she sent for her former Midwife about six of the clock in the morning, she continued in short Pains, but very sharp, till two in the Afternoon, and from that time, till nine of the clock at night, she had violent strong Pains, and very fast; and then her Midwife and Friends admitted me to be sent for. When I entered the chamber, she was just laid on the bed, and looking very fierce in my face, clapp'd her hands

hands together, in great Agony, and said, She should never be delivered; I said, I hop'd she would. I Touch'd her, but was terribly surprized, for I never found a Woman so swell'd, and was at a great stand to think how the Child could be born with safety. I turn'd to the Midwife, and ask'd her, How she could be guilty of so much cruel usage to her fellow creature? She answer'd, she knew she was very much swell'd; I told her, had it been her own case, she would have thought it very harsh usage. I proceeded to relieve the poor Woman out of her distress, and found in every Pain the Child press'd hard on the *Os Pubis*, as the former one did, when I was with her, and reliev'd her Child, and delivered her in two hours.

As soon as I had clear'd this Child from the Share-bone, I was obliged to keep it back with all my strength, three Pains, before I dar'd suffer it to be born, (for fear of ill consequences) the mother being so much swell'd. I thank God I delivered her very safe, the seventh Pain, after I was with her, and her Child was born alive, to her great Satisfaction, but was oblig'd to poultis and foment the Parts for eight days before she could turn in her bed. She recovered and did well. Her Midwife told me, that her Child had lain from seven of the clock in the morning, without any Alteration as she perceived, notwithstanding so many hours extreme Pain. I did not doubt the truth of it; but ask'd how she could expect a Delivery, as

the

the Child lay: For it was impossible it could come through the bones. I desired to know what advantage she gained by working so violently on the Woman's Body, telling her it was very detrimental to the Woman that was under her care.

When I left *Taunton*, she was with Child again, and gone half her time, and was greatly troubled at my departure.

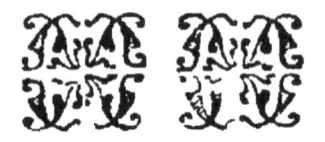

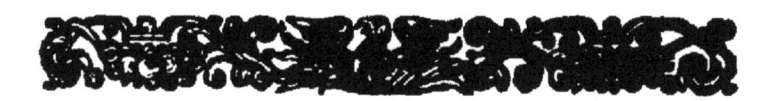

OBSERVATION XLI.

The Delivery of a Woman taken with a violent Flooding before her time.

I WAS sent for to a Gentlewoman in *Vine-street*, in *Bristol*, who was about six months gone with Child, taken with a violent Flowing of the *Menses*: 'Twas about four of the clock in the morning. I found her Physician with her, who had order'd her several Medicines, but she continued flooding very violently. I Touch'd her, but found no symptoms of Labour. I soon stopp'd her Flooding for that time,

time, and she went to sleep. I was call'd again, about eight the same morning, in great haste, her Flooding being return'd with violence. As soon as I Touch'd her, I stopp'd it again, as I have often done in my Practice, and always succeeded in ten minutes, or less, after Touching of a Woman; though it would often return again, as this Gentlewoman's did; wherefore I told her Physician it was my opinion the sooner she was delivered, the better; but he thought it best to stay, and defer it, if her Flooding did not return. But about five in the afternoon it returned; I then purposed a Delivery, though no symptoms offered but her flowing, which had caus'd the mouth of the *Matrix* to be relaxed: She desired me to deliver her; I put

I put my Fore-finger in the Mouth of the Womb, and so a second, and, by degrees, and a little strength, my whole hand; and, finding the Child lie across, I search'd for the Feet, which I soon found, and brought them forward, and so completed the Delivery in twenty minutes; and the Gentlewoman told me, she was stronger this time in one week, than she had been in three months of some of her former Children, in the same Circumstances; for she had several such before. But the only reason of her weakness, was want of a quicker Delivery, before she had lost so much Blood, as, she told me, they always suffer'd her to do, before they deliver'd her. I attended her of several Children after, at her full time, with little or no danger, more than common. I have been with many Women that have flooded prodigiously, some in Miscarriages, and some at their full time; but, thank God, I never lost any Life in that case, through all my Practice. It is a secret I would willingly have made known, for the benefit of my Sisters in the Profession: But, having a Daughter that has practised the same Art these ten years, with as good success as my self, I shall leave it in her power to make it known. There are a great many that will acknowledge, that (with the Omnipotent's leave) I have preserved the lives of many in Miscarriages; some six, seven, nay eight times miscarrying, before they have

have had a Child to live, and every time attended with violent Floodings, yet all did well.

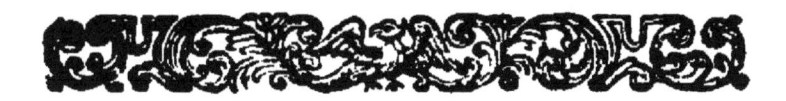

OBSERVATION XLII.

The Delivery of a Woman with the Child's Face towards the Belly.

I WAS sent for on *St. Philip's Plain*, to a Woman who had been in Pain a night and a day; but when I Touch'd her, I found her Pains were but the begining of Labour. I gave her an *Anodyne* that night, and returned home. Her Pains abated; I attended her the next day, and found but little Alteration; I ordered her the same the Night follow-

following. The next day her Pangs seemed to strengthen, but her Labour was not forward enough for my assistance; I repeated the same Draught that night. They sent for me the next morning, which was the fourth day after my first attending. I Touch'd her, and found the *Matrix* open, the breadth of a Six-pence; the Child lay very high, which was surprizing, her Pains being extreme strong: She told me they had been so violent from one of the clock in the morning, and this was about five I endeavoured to dilate the Womb, tho' to little purpose, nor could I get the Child's head off the *Os Pubis*, which did not answer my expectation, nor the poor Woman's Pains. I then suspected the Child came wrong, notwithwithstanding it presented the head first; and I desired to relinquish my place, insisting on having a Man-midwife sent for; but the Woman wou'd not suffer it, and told me, if I would not deliver her, she would die, for she'd not consent for any one else. She was a Woman of exceeding good Spirits, and did not want for Pangs, yet her Pains proved injurious to her Delivery. I again urg'd the Woman, her Mother, and Friends, to send for a Man; but they would not consent, unless I positively affirm'd I could not deliver her. I could not say that, and speak truth. I then laid her cross the bed, with a bolster and pillows under her stomach, to give the more liberty for her belly to lie hollow, that I might the better be able

able to search her, and find which way the Head came; it was with a good deal of difficulty I obtained satisfaction, by reason of the strength of her Pains. I found the Child's Face came to the Belly; it was a prodigious long-headed child, and her first, and was every way very large. I then despaired of delivering her without an Instrument, which I did not care to use: so desired them again to send for a Man-midwife; but they would not consent. I was well assured the Child could not be born with the Head foremost without an Instrument, neither could it be born unless the Child's Head was unbrain'd, with safety to the Woman; wherefore, being certain the Child was alive, I came to a Resolution to turn the Child, and

and bring it by the Feet, which I concluded would be the safest way for the Woman, but fear'd it would be too hard for the Child, yet resolv'd, with God's help, to do my duty; and so, leaving the event to the Omnipotent, I search'd for the Feet, but her Pains were so violent as to make it very difficult to get hold of a Foot; however, in about fifteen minutes, I got hold of one, and brought it towards me with all my strength; the other followed, and in half an hour, I deliver'd her of a live Child. I was greatly fatigued in turning and keeping the Face to the Back; yet had not that been done, it would not have answer'd a safe Delivery. The Woman and Child did well. I have deliver'd her of five Children since; her third Child came the same as the first, and all her Childrens Heads were prodigiously big, and very long; I was oblig'd to turn that Child also; but the Mother and Children did well.

I have had several Children come with their Faces upwards, and the Mothers have had good Times, when the Childrens Heads have been very round, and they not large. The reason of my being particular in this Observation is, having been inform'd of several Women that have been delivered with Instruments, and rent both in one, when Children have presented their Heads first, and Faces to the Belly, having long Heads; when these young Professors

fessors fixing a Hook in the poor Babe's Head, and bringing the Child off by Force (with great Strength and little Knowledge) have ruin'd many Women and Children, that I have heard of. I can speak it with sincerity, and truth, that I never injured a Woman in all my Practice, nor did I ever hear my Mother had any one such accident in all her's. Nor do I remember that I ever heard of above two, before I went to *Bristol*, that suffer'd in that manner: But the Information I have had from some Nurses, and the unfortunate Sufferers, proves it not to be very uncommon there, through mismanagement in the first beginnings of Labour; wherefore it is necessary that an exact judgment should be made,

whether

whether the Child's Head is situated right or wrong; or if the Child presses forward on the *Os Pubis*, which if it shou'd, it is best to advise the Woman to lie in her Bed, and on her Back, during her small Pains; for, by that means, her Child will settle to the Back, where it must come, before it is born. For my part, I never found when a Child was clear of the *Os Pubis*, but it would be born without pressing back the *Os Sacrum*, as is the practice of many, and, in my Judgment, without any Foundation. I have read many Authors that advise such practice, and even give directions to press back the *Os Sacrum* with all one's strength, the breadth of one's hand: Which Practice
I must

I muſt condemn, as being very prejudicial to Women; for I never found it once ſuccefsful, but very much to the contrary.

Observation XLIII.

The Delivery of a Woman, the Bottom of the Womb falling through its Neck.

I WAS ſent for to a Woman in Labour; I found her Pains very ſtrong; as ſoon as I Touch'd her, I found the Child lay right, but the Mouth of the Womb was ſunk conſiderably below the Child's Head; ſhe being in her bed, I kept her

on her Back, and, with the two fore-fingers of my right hand, I raised the Womb, and the Child came forward, and was soon born; but, to my great Suprize, going to fetch the After burden, I felt a great Substance, not unlike a Child's Head ready to be born, and finding the After-burden fast over it, I immediately supposed what it proved to be, the Bottom of the Womb fallen through its Neck, I directly put my fist against the Substance, and return'd it, but not without a good deal of strength and difficulty, and I held my hand still till I found the mouth of the Womb begin to contract itself; then I peeled off the Afterburden as you would the Rind from a Orange, and brought
it

it away with little trouble, and the Woman did very well; I kept her in bed some days longer than she used to be of her other Children, and she had not the least Complaint after, although near three months before her Delivery she complained of a great Bearing down, insomuch that she was not able to stand nor walk, but lay on a couch when out of bed, which disorder occasioned her to speak to me. She is still alive, and well, it is about four years ago, and the first and only Case of this kind I ever met with. I had not so much as Touch'd the Navel-string, when I perceiv'd this Accident; therefore the Occasion of it must proceed, as I conjecture, from the weakness of the Woman, and her

her having such a Bearing-down so long before her Labour, and the strength of her Pains, that caused the bottom of the Womb to follow the Child. The reason of my being so plain in this Observation is, that a few Years before this Accident happened to me, a Midwife was very much blam'd on account of a Woman that died in this case, in less than two hours after her Child was born, the Midwife taking the inverted Womb for another Child; and she endeavouring to deliver her, as she told her friends about her, till the Woman fainted, and then a Man-midwife was sent for; and he not being at home, they called another, and they both met near together at the Woman's man's house, but neither of them could return the Womb into its place, but they brought off the After-burden, and the Woman immediately expired.

I was informed that the Men-midwives condemned the Woman-midwife, telling her she had pulled the Navel-string with Violence, or else this Accident would not have happened; but she declared she did not; and what she said might be true; for if every Womb should be inverted by fetching the After-burden by the String, although with a considerable Strength, there would be many such accidents, which, experience tells us, seldom happen. But, I think, they would have done well, to have informed this Midwife

Midwife that, as soon as she felt the afore said substance, she should have used her art and strength to have returned it.

But, if she wanted knowledge, as I doubt she did, she should have presently sent for farther advice; for such Cases admit of no delay; therefore Midwives ought to be well instructed in every Particular of this so useful an art, for I question whether the Womb might be returned, unless it be done in a few minutes after its being inverted; for I am satisfied it was not more than four minutes after the Child was born that I was sensible of my Woman's Case, and I presently endeavoured to return the Womb; but I found

found it a difficult work; and it is not to be done without knowledge and resolution; but, praised be the Almighty God, I accomplished it.

THE END.

Lightning Source UK Ltd.
Milton Keynes UK
UKHW02f0904050418
320560UK00007B/454/P